THE GLYCEMIC INDEX MADE SIMPLE

Strategies to Lose Weight and Optimize Health

Sherry Torkos B. Sc. Phm.

John Wiley & Sons Canada, Ltd.

This book is intended for educational and informational purposes only. Please see a qualified medical professional if you have questions about your health.

The Glycemic Index Made Simple
ISBN-13: 978-0-470-84093-1

Production Credits
Cover and interior text design: Adrian So
Photo credits: Pasta: PhotoDisc/Getty Images; Strawberries: PhotoDisc/Getty Images; Bread: PhotoDisc Green/John A. Rizzo; Peppers: PhotoDisc Green/ PhotoLink
Wiley Bicentennial Logo: Richard J. Pacifico
Printer: Quebecor World

John Wiley & Sons Canada, Ltd.
6045 Freemont Blvd.
Mississauga, Ontario, L5R 4J3
Printed in the United States

1 2 3 4 5 QW0 11 10 09 08 07

Contents

Acknowledgements

There are many people who I would like to acknowledge and thank for their help in this book.

My partner Rick for all your support and encouragement throughout this book project and all the others over the years.

To my developmental editor Kate Zia, I can't thank you enough for all your guidance and assistance with all aspects of this book. It is a pleasure working with you.

To the team at John Wiley & Sons: Christiane Cote, Leah Fairbank, Liz Mc-Curdy, and Jennifer Smith, I thank you for this opportunity, and your literary guidance and expertise throughout the entire process.

A special thanks to my colleagues, Mitch Skop, Dean Mosca, Tom McCartney and Mike Danielson for all your support in this book and the many other projects that we have worked on together.

I would also like to acknowledge the many researchers that have worked so hard to help us understand obesity, weight loss, and the role of glycemic control:

Thomas Wolever, DM, PhD, David J.A. Jenkins, MD, Jenny Brand-Miller, PhD, PhD, DSc, Harry Preuss, MD, and Jay Udani, MD.

Dedication

I dedicate this book to all those people struggling with their weight and interested in improving their health. It is my sincere hope that this book empowers you on your journey to optimum health.

Foreword
by Harry Preuss, MD, MACN, CNS

By now, most of us understand that being overweight is not just an appearance issue, or about the inconvenience of having many different clothing sizes in your closet. As a medical practitioner; professor of physiology, medicine and pathology; and researcher in the field of obesity and weight loss, I can attest to obesity's power to destroy one's health and quality of life—both mentally and physically.

It is generally recognized that being obese predisposes an individual to diabetes mellitus, coronary artery disease, stroke, sleep apnea, degenerative joint disease, and most likely certain forms of cancer. In January 2004, the *Journal of Obesity Research* published a study co-authored by the CDC that estimated that U.S. obesity-attributable medical expenditures reached $75 billion in 2003 and that taxpayers financed about half of these costs through Medicare and Medicaid. Therefore, I applaud Sherry's commitment to educating the public about this very serious health issue. Clearly we must take action if we want to live well.

While many fad diets promise miraculous results, unfortunately, far too many are based on hype rather than science. Dietary changes are critical, but there are other factors to consider. A balanced approach to weight loss includes several lifestyle modifications in addition to dietary regimens—exercise (both aerobic and anaerobic), avoidance of stress, and adequate sleep. This book pulls it all together and appeals not only to those trying to lose weight but also to those interested in improving their health and cutting their risk of chronic disease.

A low glycemic diet that lessens the load of rapidly absorbed carbohydrates is a healthy way of eating, because it is associated with better blood sugar control, superior health, and improved weight management. Like the majority of Americans, I love good food, and I can confirm that an eating style that improves the glycemic load is not restrictive or hard to follow. It incorporates reasonable portions of fresh, whole, unprocessed foods that possess healthful nutrients.

Why worry about rapidly rising blood sugar concentrations? Too much sugar rising in the circulation from poor dietary choices is associated with insulin resistance, which can lead to all sorts of health problems, including diabetes. Accordingly, controlling rapid elevations in blood sugar can reduce your risk of several chronic diseases, and even slow the advance of symptoms associated with aging.

Gaining control of your blood sugar also helps reduce appetite and cravings for sweets, and enhances energy levels.

The glycemic index and the glycemic load are new tools that help us understand how carbohydrates impact blood sugar. It is worth repeating that numerous studies have linked diets high in the glycemic load to obesity, and increased risk factors for heart disease, diabetes and cancer. On the other hand, low glycemic index and load diets have been shown to help protect against these conditions.

This book will help you make the transition to better health by educating you on the rationale behind the glycemic index and glycemic load for weight loss and overall health, teaching you how to make healthy low glycemic food choices, and giving you simple strategies for incorporating a low glycemic diet into your daily life. You will also find information on other factors that influence weight, and advice on how to improve these aspects of your life. From advice on supplements that can help improve blood sugar control and aid weight loss to tips on making adjustments in all aspects of your life, Sherry empowers you to make the necessary lifestyle changes that will enable you to live a higher quality of life.

Harry Preuss, MD, MACN, CNS, is a tenured professor at Georgetown Medical Center. His current research centers on the use of dietary supplements and nutraceuticals to favorably influence or even prevent obesity, insulin resistance, and heart disease. The author of hundreds of medical papers and abstracts, he is co-author of The Prostate Cure *(Crown, 1998) and the upcoming book entitled* The Natural Fat Loss Pharmacy *(Broadway Book, 2007). He lives in Fairfax Station, Virginia.*

Introduction

Not Another Diet Book

If I were a betting woman, I'd bet this book caught your eye because you've struggled to lose weight and heard the glycemic index was the latest diet phenomenon. But, if you're looking for a diet that can provide rapid weight loss, I'm afraid you've got the wrong book. While following the glycemic index has been shown to reduce weight and decrease body fat over time, the diet is more about a way to have good health rather than a quick fix along the road. The story of the glycemic index is not about the latest diet touted by celebrities; it's about making good food choices everyday that will improve blood sugar regulation and ultimately yield long-term health benefits.

Eating according to the glycemic index is based on science and physiology, geared for those willing to commit to their lifelong health. It is for those people who are aware of the profound effects of blood sugar imbalances, and want to do something about it before those imbalances turn into chronic disease. So, this is not another diet book. But if you take the time to learn about the glycemic index, and make the necessary changes to your diet and lifestyle, you will be pleased with the results. While you may not have found the quick-fix diet you thought you wanted, you did find the healthy diet you need to reach your weight-loss goals and improve your health. It's all about winning at weight loss, and I believe the glycemic index is the ideal tool to help you succeed.

Glycemic Index: Short and Sweet

First introduced in the 1980s by Canadian researchers, the glycemic index or GI is a system of ranking all forms of carbohydrates (breads, rice, legumes, fruits and vegetables) on a scale of zero to one hundred on how they affect blood glucose levels and consequently insulin levels. If a carbohydrate is digested quickly and causes a rapid rise in blood sugar levels, it is considered to be "high GI." If a carbohydrate is more slowly digested and causes a gentle rise in blood sugar levels, it is considered "low GI." Research indicates that by choosing carbohydrates that are low GI as well as healthy (very important!), people may experience significant weight loss as well as decreased body fat. By keeping blood sugar levels balanced, people also experience balanced moods, reduced hunger cravings, and increased metabolic rate—all important factors to promote long-term weight loss and weight management. Plus, a low GI diet has been found to reduce the risk of diabetes and heart disease, which are two of the biggest health threats we face today.

Is THE GLYCEMIC INDEX RIGHT FOR ME?

The glycemic index is not a diet in the typical sense of that word. It is a guide for making healthy carbohydrate choices much like the daily food-serving guides we see at schools or the doctor's office. If you follow the glycemic index, you will still eat a balanced and varied selection of carbohydrates, along with quality proteins and healthy fats. There are no food combining rules to memorize, no calorie counting and no depriving yourself of a particular food group. Your food consumption is not restricted beyond eating healthy portion sizes, and there are absolutely no missed meals. The glycemic index can be followed by people of all ages, and does not cause any adverse effects, like some of the fad diets. Under a doctor's supervision, even people with existing health concerns such as Type 2 diabetes or heart disease can follow a diet based on the glycemic index. In fact, there are significant health benefits to eating according to the glycemic index because it not only helps combat obesity and diabetes, two conditions at nearly epidemic proportions, but also addresses a growing health concern today: insulin resistance.

A MESSY LOVE TRIANGLE: BLOOD SUGAR, INSULIN AND YOUR WEIGHT

To understand how the glycemic index can improve health, first we need to understand the connection between blood sugar, insulin and body weight. As blood sugar, or blood glucose rises, the body produces insulin to transport it into the cells to be used as energy. If blood sugar levels remain high or dramatically fluctuate throughout the day then insulin production will do the same. Overtime, the body can become resistant to the effects of insulin, a condition called insulin resistance, and both blood sugar and insulin levels remain high.

It is estimated that over twenty-five percent of the population worldwide has insulin resistance. Not only does this dramatically increase the risk of developing Type 2 diabetes and heart disease, but insulin resistance is also at the root of the phenomenon known as metabolic syndrome. Unfortunately, because there are often no evident symptoms of insulin resistance it goes undiagnosed and therefore untreated for years and even decades.

Insulin resistance is now recognized as a major contributor to obesity. There are many reasons for this. When insulin levels are high, the body stores more fat, we have stronger appetites and food cravings, and our bodies release more cortisol, which causes fat to accumulate around the mid-section. Belly fat is now known to produce chemicals that stimulate inflammation and worsen insulin sensitivity. So as you can see, controlling insulin levels through a low GI diet, can play a vital role in weight management.

It is a common misconception that only those with diabetes need to worry about their blood sugar. Blood sugar regulation is an important part of overall health. Many years ago blood sugar may not have been a mainstream concern but today, with the typical diet including massive amounts of refined carbohydrates and sugar-rich foods, even those without diabetes are developing concerns related to blood sugar. However, through regular exercise and a healthy, low-glycemic diet, you can successfully balance blood sugar and decrease insulin levels throughout the day, thereby reducing your risk of insulin resistance and its resulting health problems.

How to Use this Book: Just the Facts Please

I've written this book to provide you with a thorough explanation of the role of the glycemic index in weight loss, disease prevention and optimal health. I've made the science as reader-friendly as possible, referenced current research and provided the best resources for you to refer to when deciding if the glycemic index is right for you.

I start the book with an overview of the worldwide obesity epidemic and its impact on health. I discuss the problems associated with fad diets and our obsession with weight. I explore the causes of obesity and factors affecting body weight, and provide information on how to determine your ideal weight.

You'll then find a complete description of the glycemic index and how it to follow it. You'll learn about the glycemic load, and read about international research projects from the past, and on-going studies from today, which underscore the medical importance of choosing low-glycemic carbohydrates. You'll find a thorough description of diabetes and the role of insulin and insulin resistance. There are descriptions of how blood sugar affects appetite and mood, weight, aging and heart health. I've also included information on the role of the other important macronutrients for health, energy and weight control, namely proteins and fats.

You will then learn how to include the glycemic index with a broader health and diet strategy. I outline my recommended principles for following the glycemic index and include a glycemic index food values chart. You will learn about the role of functional foods and water for weight management and overall health. I also go through two newly recognized factors that affect weight—stress and lack of sleep—and why these two factors are so critical for lifelong health. And lastly, I outline my recommendations for supplements that support blood sugar regulation and weight loss.

Lastly, readers will get advice on how to roll up their sleeves, take what they've learned and put it into action. I discuss overcoming the obstacles to following a low-GI diet, particularly during holidays and when dining out. You'll find a seven-day diet plan with meal recommendations to get you started in the right direction.

THE GLYCEMIC INDEX IS HERE TO STAY

When I wrote my book *Winning at Weight Loss* in 2002, the glycemic index existed but it was not a commonly heard phrase. Today, many people have heard of the glycemic index but still don't understand it properly, and how it can impact their health. The glycemic index is growing in popularity and, through science, becoming widely accepted as a beneficial way of eating. Today doctors, dietitians and other health care practitioners recommend the glycemic index for patients with weight or diabetic concerns, and for those looking to optimize health.

In the past decade, the glycemic index has been the subject of substantial research. Our understanding of the glycemic index and how it benefits weight loss and blood sugar balancing has increased substantially. There is significant research being done around the world to bring the glycemic index to the mainstream not as a fad diet but as a legitimate style of eating—for better health. The goal of this book is to make information about eating according to the glycemic index accessible to you.

1

CHAPTER

The Obesity Epidemic

Our society is bombarded by a tremendous amount of information on research and developments in the area of lifestyle, fitness and nutrition. Yet, we're slow to put that good information into action in our personal lives. Around the world, chronic disease, frequently brought about by lifestyle factors, threatens us all. Heart disease remains the number one killer of men and women in Western societies. Diabetes impacts an estimated two million Canadians and twenty-one million Americans. Within the next decade, osteoarthritis is predicted to become a leading cause of disability. Experts agree that these diseases are largely preventable; however, often it is not until we are diagnosed with a particular condition that we feel motivated enough to do something about it. This apathy toward our long-term health is nowhere more apparent than when it comes to weight and the global obesity epidemic. Consider this stunning statistic: *there is an estimated one billion people classed as either overweight or obese around the world.*

Change is not easy, especially when it comes to lifestyle factors such as diet and exercise. With our fast paced way of living, priorities get mislaid and we don't take time for sleep, proper eating and regular exercise—elements required for a healthy body. Sadly, despite the attention given to the obesity epidemic, we are not making much progress. Rates are continuing to soar, affecting younger and younger people, and bringing on chronic disease and premature death.

OBESITY STATISTICS CAN NO LONGER BE IGNORED

Currently, in the United States over sixty percent of adults are overweight, with thirty percent classified as obese. These figures represent an increase of more than fifty percent in the last ten years alone. Direct medical costs as a result are at an astounding 105 billion dollars, or nine percent of the nation's health care costs.

In Canada, obesity rates are up in almost every age group, with a notable increase in children and adolescents. According to the 2004 Canadian Community Health Survey, eight percent of children ages twelve to seventeen are obese, compared to three percent in the 1978/79 survey. In the same time frame, adult obesity rates have nearly doubled from fourteen percent to twenty-three percent; that represents 5.5 million Canadians struggling not just with excess weight, but also with obesity. This health epidemic translates into an estimated five billion dollar burden on the Canadian economy. And while both men and women are equally likely to be obese, the survey found a higher percentage of women were classed in the most severe category of obesity, significantly increasing their risk of developing chronic diseases. Statistics indicate that obese individuals have a fifty to one hundred percent likelihood of dying prematurely due to chronic disease caused by obesity.

Obesity is no longer just a Western disease. International rates are also on the rise. According to the 2004 OECD Health Data report (*Organization for Economic Co-Operation and Development*), in the twenty-nine countries that participate in this organization, obesity rates have significantly increased in the past two decades, with the average obesity rate currently sitting at thirteen percent of the adult population. Japan and Korea had the lowest obesity rates at approximately three percent while the United States was the highest with thirty percent. The United Kingdom, Australia, New Zealand, Canada and Mexico all reported obesity rates of over twenty percent.

- In the United Kingdom, obesity rates have quadrupled in the last twenty-five years, with three-quarters of the population overweight and an estimated twenty-two percent classed as obese. The childhood obesity rate has tripled in the last twenty years. Over thirty thousand deaths are attributed to obesity, costing the nation over seven billion pounds per year in health care and related costs.
- In Australia, obesity rates have more than doubled in the past twenty years. While the rate is lower than North America, with approximately forty-eight percent of the population classed as overweight or obese the Australian Institute of Health and Welfare predicts that number to grow to by more than twelve percent by 2010.
- In New Zealand, one-third of the adult population is overweight and one-fifth of the adult population is obese, according to a New Zealand Ministry of Health report in 2003.
- In Mexico, obesity rates are one of the highest in the world with over sixty percent overweight or obese in 1999 (up from thirty-three percent in 1988). One report indicated that obesity rates might rise as high as eighty-five percent of women and seventy-five percent of men. Infectious disease no longer accounts for as many causes of death as cardiovascular disease and diabetes, which are directly associated with obesity.

CHILDHOOD OBESITY

Sadly, young people represent the largest growing segment of the obese population. According to an estimate by the International Obesity Task Force, twenty-two million of the world's children five years and younger are overweight or obese. According to a study conducted by the California Department of Health Services, eighty percent of children have been on a diet by the time they have reached the fourth grade. In the United States, obesity rates in children have almost tripled in the past twenty-five years. The picture is worse in Canada. A long-term study of Canadian children revealed one of the highest rates of childhood obesity in the world. At least one in four is overweight, compared to one in ten when the study began in 1981. Unfortunately, this trend is also being seen in other areas of the world such as Europe, Australia and the Caribbean.

The obesity epidemic is having far-reaching effects on the health of our children. A recent study found one in eight children have three or more risk factors for metabolic syndrome, a cluster of symptoms that serve as an early warning signal for heart disease and diabetes. And more than half of these children have at least one of the risk factors. These risk factors include high blood pressure, inefficient processing of glucose, elevated insulin levels, low levels of "good" HDL cholesterol and elevated triglycerides.

Overweight children are at risk of becoming obese adults, and obese adults are at greater risk for raising obese children. While genetics are often blamed, in many cases it is poor lifestyle habits that are inherited rather than faulty genes.

RESEARCH SPOTLIGHT: "CHILDREN DEVELOPING POT-BELLIES"

Led by researchers at the US Centers for Disease Control, a recent study published in *Pediatrics* reports that abdominal obesity in American children increased more than sixty-five percent among boys and almost seventy percent among girls between 1988 and 2004. This was startling news because studies have shown the increased risk of heart disease and Type 2 diabetes due to excess body fat is mainly due to belly fat. While the study reported an overall increase in body mass index in children from youngsters to teens, what worried experts was the significant increases in abdominal or belly fat. The good news is that, for children and adolescents, the health effects from excess belly fat are often reversible through changes to diet and lifestyle.

OBESITY'S IMPACT ON HEALTH

It is hard to escape the warnings from our national health agencies. The message they deliver is clear: obesity increases the risk of developing chronic disease. Just like smoking, obesity is one of the most preventable causes of chronic disease because in most cases its development is lifestyle-related. Taking in too many calories, eating unhealthy foods and not getting enough exercise are lifestyle choices,

"Obesity's impact is so diverse and extreme that it should now be regarded as one of the greatest neglected public health problems of our time, with an impact on health which may well prove to be as great as that of smoking."

—World Health Organization

choices that can lead to serious consequences. These are not the only factors that affect our weight, but they are the major ones. Some of the other elements that affect body weight are discussed in a later section.

One of the most serious consequences of being overweight is the increased risk of heart disease. Carrying excess weight increases blood pressure because the heart has to work harder and becomes strained. Having elevated blood pressure, known as hypertension, increases the risk of coronary heart disease and stroke.

Those who are overweight also tend to develop high cholesterol and there are several reasons for this. First, dietary factors can raise cholesterol—eating a diet high in saturated and trans fats can raise cholesterol levels and overeating can raise triglycerides. Second, overweight individuals are at risk for developing insulin resistance, a condition where the body becomes resistant to the effects of insulin so that insulin and blood sugar levels remain high. When insulin levels are high the liver increases triglyceride production which lowers HDL (good) cholesterol and increases LDL (bad) cholesterol. This combination of factors can substantially increase the risk of heart disease.

Studies also show that overweight people are more susceptible to breast and colon cancers. Other health risks associated with obesity include post-surgical complications, delayed wound healing and an increased risk of infection and gout. Excess weight can put pressure on your lungs and chest, making it difficult to breathe and causing sleep apnea. It can also be stressful to the joints, back and hips leading to osteoarthritis, limited mobility, pain and discomfort. Overweight and obese women are at greater risk of having infertility and complications during childbirth.

DIABESITY: THE UNION OF OBESITY AND DIABETES

One of the most talked about consequences of obesity is the development of diabetes. In fact researchers have coined a term for this association: *diabesity*. According to a report from the Centers for Disease Control, diabetes has officially reached epidemic proportions. The link between obesity and diabetes is quite strong—over sixty percent of people with Type 2 diabetes are obese. Researchers agree, the more weight you carry, the greater your chances of suffering from diabetes and other blood sugar related conditions. This information should be taken as an incentive to take action on weight concerns.

WHAT'S LIFESTYLE GOT TO DO WITH IT?

It seems to go without saying that the likelihood of being overweight or obese is related to diet and exercise. According to the 2004 Canadian Community Health Survey, adult men and women who ate fruit and vegetables less than three times a day were more likely to be obese than were those who consumed such foods five or more times a day. This is not surprising because when unhealthy foods (fast food, processed foods) take the place of healthy foods, such as fruits and vegetables, calorie intake increases and blood sugar regulation is impaired, both of which cause weight gain. Similarly, people who spent their leisure time in sedentary pursuits rather than being physically active were more likely to be obese: twenty-seven percent of sedentary men were obese, compared with twenty percent of active men. Among women, obesity rates were high not only for those who were sedentary, but also for those who were moderately active.

OBSESSED WITH WEIGHT...

Certainly, obesity is a profound medical problem facing society. Those with excess body fat need to slim down for better heart health, a lower risk of certain cancers and diabetes, fewer symptoms of osteoarthritis and a host of other health benefits. While it is clearly documented that being overweight is a risk factor for many chronic diseases, being overweight also has far-reaching effects on a person's self-esteem, confidence and overall emotional well-being. Struggling with your weight and dieting can have a profound effect on quality of life, triggering anxiety, depression and an often-overwhelming sense of failure and hopelessness. However, the other extreme—being seriously underweight—is just as dangerous, increasing the risk of osteoporosis and damage to the heart and other organs.

Finding a healthy balance in today's world isn't easy. It doesn't help that our culture has become obsessed with celebrity and bodily perfection. In the last five years alone, there has been a distinct shift regarding weight and body shape. Women now feel a tremendous social pressure to achieve stick-thin figures at any cost. Young starlets are admonished for their frighteningly unhealthy frames and yet simultaneously rewarded with countless magazine covers for their efforts. Many young women today have turned to caffeine, nicotine and other more addictive and destructive drugs such as "crystal meth" to achieve this idealized skeletal frame. The message is clear: be thin or be nothing.

This detrimental message has resulted in an increase in eating disorders, for men and women of all ages. According to some reports, one in three dieters develop compulsive eating disorders while one in four will develop full-blown eating disorders, such as anorexia or bulimia. An estimated one percent of American females suffer from anorexia nervosa, a potentially life-threatening illness characterized by excessive dieting, depression and extreme weight loss. In the United States, an estimated two percent of college students and one percent of women in general suffer from bulimia nervosa (bingeing and purging). Bulimia is associated with health problems such as tears in the stomach lining, ruptures, irregular heartbeat, kidney damage from potassium deficiency, damaged tooth enamel and cessation of menstrual periods.

Although ninety to ninety-five percent of people with eating disorders such as anorexia and bulimia are women, these conditions also affect men. In fact, men account for up to forty percent of those with compulsive eating behaviours. The factors that predispose men to eating disorders are similar to those that affect women:

- A history of being overweight or dieting;
- Involvement in activities where thinness is important, such as dance, gymnastics, running, track and field, horseback riding, wrestling and body building;
- Involvement in careers that value thinness, such as fashion, modelling and acting, and
- Living among people who equate thinness with attractiveness and value.

Considering the ultra-thin images that bombard us from television, movies and magazines, it is no wonder people—especially young women—feel fat even though they are not. The typical model is between five feet, eight inches and five feet, ten inches tall and weighs 120 pounds. Even though her knee joints may be wider than her thighs, her skinny frame is what many women seek. In contrast, the average North American woman is five feet, four inches tall and weighs 138 pounds. Approximately one out of every forty thousand women has a "model-perfect" body. Clearly, this is an unrealistic and unhealthy ideal for the vast majority of women. Interestingly, Marilyn Monroe, the pinup girl for the 1950s, wore a size fourteen, and I think we all agree that she was gorgeous.

And yet, today two out of five women say they would trade up to five years *of their lives* to achieve their ideal body type. It is clear that the obsession has become solely focused on weight and the benefits of achieving a healthy body weight have been forgotten in the process. Is this the message we want to continue to convey to the next generation of women? Many organizations are saying a loud "NO." In the fall of 2006, Spain banned "ultra-thin" models from fashion catwalks, triggering dialogue about the issue. Dove beauty products' Campaign for Real Beauty, which features real women instead of models in their advertisements, has struck a chord for many women, inspiring a six hundred percent increase in sales in the first two months of its launch and a short film series exploring the social issues surrounding our obsession with weight.

...And Desperately Dieting

The prevalence of obesity is a paradox in our thinness-obsessed Western culture. As a result, North Americans spend billions in an effort to slim down. It is estimated that North Americans spend more than forty-six billion dollars annually on weight-loss products and services. Weight Watchers, established in 1961, now totals annual sales at over one billion dollars. There are endless programs, products and diet pills on the market. It is estimated that more than six billion dollars is spent yearly on diet pills alone. The concern here is that many of these products do not work. Very few diet pills have been clinically tested, and some may even be hazardous to your health. Furthermore, when dieters do lose weight, they usually gain it back, according to a panel of obesity, metabolic and other experts, who were convened by the National Institutes of Health (NIH). Studies show that one year after dieting, sixty-six percent of people regain any lost weight. Government findings report that after five years, ninety-seven percent of dieters regained all the weight they had lost. Maintaining weight loss is even more difficult than losing it because it takes a long-term commitment to a lifestyle that involves healthy eating and regular exercise. Slipping back to old habits is hard to resist.

FAD DIETS ARE NOT THE ANSWER

Despite the failure and frustration of fad diets, we get enticed by the sensational advertisements and are keen to hear about and try the newest weight-loss miracle. Each week there seems to be a new diet program or plan promoted in the tabloids. Promises for quick results and celebrity endorsements give us false hope and the belief that these plans will work for us. Unfortunately many of these diets are not backed by science, and some can be dangerous to your health. For example, a recent diet I came across promotes that you can lose ten pounds in two days by consuming a liquid tonic of various herbs and nutrients. No food is allowed, or any liquids other than water for the two days. No doubt, a two-day fast will result in some weight loss. Since the product contains herbs with diuretic properties, water loss will also occur. Yet, I highly doubt this product will deliver on its claims. Interestingly, the company did not have any studies to back up their claims, and only a handful of dubious testimonials. It is important to realize that rapid weight loss that occurs from fasting or taking diuretics and laxatives is temporary and can be dangerous, especially for those with diabetes, or kidney or heart problems. Once you start eating and drinking fluids again, the weight will come back.

Stay away from diets that are drastically low in calories (less than eight hundred calories per day). While these diets can lead to rapid weight loss, they are not without risks. Low calorie diets cause the body to cannibalize (break down) its own muscle for fuel, causing muscle-wasting, which reduces metabolism. Plus these diets can induce nutrient deficiencies, fatigue, compromised immune function, and over the long term, may result in starvation, organ failure and death.

BMI HELPS ESTABLISH HEALTHY WEIGHTS

There are a variety of methods used to determine whether you are carrying excess weight and are at risk of developing health problems. The easiest and most common method is the body mass index (BMI). The BMI is a mathematical formula that is highly correlated with body fat and which has gained international acceptance.

The BMI represents your weight in pounds, divided by your height in inches squared. Here is how you calculate it in imperial measurements:

1. Multiply your weight, in pounds, by 0.45
2. Multiply your height, in inches, by 0.025
3. Square the answer from step 2
4. Divide the answer from step 1 by the answer from step 3

For example, if you weigh 140 pounds and are five feet, six inches tall (66 inches), your BMI would be calculated as follows:

1. 140 pounds x 0.45 = 63
2. 66 inches x 0.025 = 1.65
3. 1.65 x 1.65 = 2.72
4. 63 divided by 2.72 = 23.16

BODY MASS INDEX

BMI (kg/m2)	19	20	21	22	23	24	25	26	27	28	29	30	35	40
Height (inches)	Weight in pounds													
58	91	96	100	105	110	115	119	124	129	134	138	143	167	191
59	94	99	104	109	114	119	124	128	133	138	143	148	173	198
60	97	102	107	112	118	123	128	133	138	143	148	153	179	204
61	100	106	111	116	122	127	132	137	143	148	153	158	185	211
62	104	109	115	120	126	131	136	142	147	153	158	164	191	218
63	107	113	118	124	130	135	141	146	152	158	163	169	197	225
64	110	116	122	128	134	140	145	151	157	163	169	174	204	232
65	114	120	126	132	138	144	150	156	162	168	174	180	210	240
66	118	124	130	136	142	148	155	161	167	173	179	186	216	247
67	121	127	134	140	146	153	159	166	172	178	185	191	223	255
68	125	131	138	144	151	158	164	171	177	184	190	197	230	262
69	128	135	142	149	155	162	169	176	182	189	196	203	236	270
70	132	139	146	153	160	167	174	181	188	195	202	207	243	278
71	136	143	150	157	165	172	179	186	193	200	208	215	250	286
72	140	147	154	162	169	177	184	191	199	206	213	221	258	294
73	144	151	159	166	174	182	189	197	204	212	219	227	265	302
74	148	155	163	171	179	186	194	202	210	218	225	233	272	311
75	152	160	168	176	184	192	200	208	216	224	232	240	279	319
76	156	164	172	180	189	197	205	213	221	230	238	246	287	328

If your BMI is under 18.5, you may be underweight. If your BMI falls between 18.5 and 24.9—as is the case in the previous example—your weight is likely within normal range. If your BMI is over twenty-five, you are probably overweight. If it is over thirty, you are likely obese.

A drawback of the BMI is that it neither distinguishes fat from muscle, nor takes into account the higher body fat content normally found in females. Because body composition (fat versus muscle) is a more important factor in determining health risks, it is also important to check your percentage of body fat. This can be done by a variety of methods:

- Bioelectric Impedance—a machine is used to measure an electric signal as it passes through lean body mass and fat. The higher the fat content the greater the resistance to the current.
- Near Infrared Technology—infrared light is shined on to the skin (usually bicep area). Fat absorbs the light, while lean body mass reflects the lights back. The reflected light is measured by a special sensor, transmitted into the computer, and translated into percentage of body fat. This method is highly accurate and is available at health centers and gyms.
- DEXA—stands for dual energy X-ray absorptiometry. X-ray energies are used to measure body fat, muscle and bone mineral. This method is highly accurate but also the most expensive and time consuming.

Men with more than twenty-five percent and women with more than thirty percent body fat are considered to be obese. The target body fat range for women is fifteen to twenty-five percent, and for men it is ten to twenty percent.

FINDING A HEALTHY BALANCE

Being either too fat or too thin creates health problems. Obesity is by far the greatest health dilemma in North American society, but it is important not to go overboard in the other direction. For example, if you are a five feet, ten inches tall man and you weigh 165 pounds, your BMI is twenty-four—within normal range. You may not fit into the jeans you wore in high school, but you probably do not need to lose weight. Keep eating right, exercise consistently to keep your muscle mass and make sure your BMI stays under twenty-five. If you are a woman five feet, four inches tall, and you weigh 135 pounds, your BMI is twenty-three, which is fine. You may not resemble super model Kate Moss, but you can stand your ground in a strong wind.

For middle-aged women, gaining a few pounds may have a protective function. One theory is that women tend to gain some weight around menopause because their bodies are trying to hang on to estrogen, which is stored in fat tissue. A forty-five-year-old woman should not expect to have the same figure she had when she was sixteen, but she also needs to stay within a healthy BMI. If her weight is too low, she may increase her risk of osteoporosis; if her weight is too high, she becomes more susceptible to diabetes, heart disease, stroke and certain cancers.

Health authorities agree that in order to maintain long-term weight loss, you need to make long-term changes to your lifestyle. I can't stress enough how important a proper diet and regular physical activity are for weight management and overall health. A large piece of the puzzle will be to let go of the obsession with weight and focus on the benefits that come from a healthy lifestyle. With these long-term changes you will reap great health benefits—greater energy and vitality, and a reduced risk of chronic disease. To reach and maintain a healthy weight, learn to make critical distinctions between weight loss and fat loss, between diet and nutrition, and between being thin and being healthy.

UNDERSTANDING THE FACTORS THAT CONTRIBUTE TO OBESITY

In the past, the first law of thermodynamics was often used to explain the control of body weight. Simply put, if energy intake (food) exceeds energy expenditures (exercise/activity), then weight gain occurs. Conversely, reducing intake and increasing expenditures was believed to be the key to weight loss. For years, doctors and researchers believed this simple theory to be the answer. We now know, however, that other factors are involved. Some people can exercise religiously, reduce food intake and still not lose weight. And, of course, we all know people who can eat whatever they want and never gain a pound. Weight gain and obesity are complex conditions, dependent upon various lifestyle, hormonal, biochemical, metabolic and genetic factors. Some of the most important factors include the following:

- Basal Metabolic Rate (BMR)—your BMR is the rate at which your body burns calories at rest. This rate is dependent on several of the factors listed below, such as activity level and thyroid function.
- Caloric Intake—overeating and consuming more calories than your body uses for energy can result in weight gain, regardless of whether those calories come from fat, carbohydrates or protein.
- Physical activity—our activity level is the major player in weight balance. Inactivity causes loss of muscle mass, a reduced metabolic rate and increased body fat. Conversely, regular exercise can improve muscle mass and boost metabolism. As we exercise, our muscles utilize calories for energy and generate heat, which promotes the burning of fat.
- Quality of food—eating too much saturated fat, sugar, processed food and fast food is associated with weight gain. Eating foods that trigger blood sugar imbalances (high glycemic foods) is also associated with weight gain and an inability to lose weight.
- Stress—exposure to chronic stress can cause weight gain, particularly around the mid-section. This occurs because stress increases the production and release of cortisol, a hormone that increases fat storage (particularly around the belly).

- Lack of sleep—insufficient sleep, even for as short a period as a week, can trigger hormonal imbalances such as decreased sensitivity to insulin and decreased production of leptin and serotonin (factors that trigger appetite). Lack of sleep also increases the production of the hormone ghrelin, which increases appetite.
- Genetics—genetics may be responsible for about twenty-five percent of obesity cases, but experts agree that having a genetic predisposition towards obesity does not mean that this is your fate. Several studies have shown that lifestyle factors are more important determinants.
- Hormones and Brain Chemicals:

  – Insulin: when insulin levels are high, the body stores more fat and is not able to use fat as a source of energy, which is the reason insulin is also known as "the fat storage hormone." This can be a problem for those with insulin resistance who often develop hyperinsulinemia (high insulin levels).
  – Thyroid: the thyroid gland plays a vital role in controlling metabolism. If your thyroid is sluggish and not functioning optimally, this can reduce your metabolic rate and cause weight gain.
  – Leptin: satiety is also regulated by leptin, a hormone produced by body fat. Researchers have found that some people become resistant to their own leptin. To compensate for this, the body produces more and more of the hormone, but the "satisfied" message is not properly received by the brain.
  – Serotonin: serotonin is a chemical messenger in the brain that regulates satiety. When levels are low, we feel hungry and when they are high, we feel satisfied. Certain weight-loss products work by elevating serotonin to promote satiety and reduce cravings for food.
  – Human Growth Hormone (HGH): by increasing lean muscle mass and reducing body fat storage, human growth hormone regulates body weight. Levels decline with age, particularly after age fifty, causing a shift in our body composition. As HGH decreases, we gain body fat and lose muscle mass.
  – Estrogen: high estrogen levels are associated with weight gain. Yet, many women find that they gain weight during menopause while their estrogen levels are lower. This happens because as estrogen levels decline in menopause, as a compensatory mechanism, the fat cells take over the production of estrogen. In order to meet the growing demand during menopause, the fat cells increase in size and number.
  – Testosterone: testosterone helps the body maintain lean muscle mass and burn fat. A deficiency of this hormone can cause the loss of muscle mass and fat gain. This is a significant contributor to fat gain in older men.

LOSE WEIGHT AND LIVE LONGER

Controlling your weight may extend your lifespan. In a study published in the *Journal of the American Medical Association*, researchers looked at body weight and mortality in a group of 19,000 middle-aged men over the course of twenty-seven years. Researchers found that the men who were lean lived significantly longer than those who were extremely under- or overweight. This is no surprise, considering the effects that excess weight has on your risk of developing chronic disease.

Research in women has yielded the same results. A study published in the May 2004 issue of the *Journal of the American Medical Association* found that both obesity and physical activity significantly and independently affected mortality. This study involved over 115,000 women who were followed for twenty-four years. Compared to physically active, lean women, there was nearly a two-and-a-half-fold increase in risk of death for inactive and obese women. The researchers estimated that excess weight (BMI over twenty-five) and physical inactivity (less than 3.5 hours per week) accounted for thirty-one percent of all premature deaths among the study participants with fifty-nine percent of the deaths attributable to cardiovascular disease and twenty-one percent from cancer among the non-smoking women. The researchers concluded, "It is clear that both weight and exercise are important for health and longevity. There is no question that you should be as active as possible no matter what your weight is, but it is equally important to maintain a healthy weight and prevent weight gain through diet and lifestyle."

We can't afford to ignore the health consequences of obesity. We need to take steps now to adopt a healthier lifestyle. Keep in mind that even small losses lead to great health rewards. If you are overweight, losing even five to ten percent of that excess weight can dramatically improve your health by lowering your blood pressure, cholesterol level and blood sugar. Plus, you will have more energy, sleep better and enjoy better overall health.

Researchers continually seek a greater understanding of obesity so they can develop more effective strategies for treating it. In the meantime, we must realize that there is no "magic bullet" for weight loss. Instead, we need to develop a comprehensive strategy that includes a balanced diet, consistent exercise and safe supplementation.

—∿—

By now you should have a more thorough understanding of obesity, the importance of healthy weight loss and healthy attitudes towards our bodies, as well as the factors that contribute to weight gain. Let's now take an in-depth look at how and why balancing blood sugar and the glycemic index are gaining momentum as revolutionary concepts to incorporate into a weight management strategy.

2
CHAPTER

Just What Is the Glycemic Index?

The glycemic index (GI) is a tool that can help people lose weight and decrease their risk or manage their symptoms of diabetes and cardiovascular disease. It is a scale that measures how quickly carbohydrates are broken down into sugar (also called blood sugar or blood glucose), which is used as "fuel" by the cells in the body. Those carbohydrates that are rapidly digested and broken down into blood glucose are ranked as "high GI." These include simple carbohydrates such as sugar and refined starches such as white bread. Those carbohydrates that are more slowly digested and broken down into blood glucose have a "low GI," including most vegetables, non-tropical fruits and unprocessed grains.

Eating high GI foods can lead to blood sugar imbalances, which may result in fatigue, increased appetite and increased food cravings, particularly for sweets. Furthermore, numerous studies have linked diets that include large amounts of high GI foods to obesity, increased belly fat, insulin resistance, Type 2 diabetes, high cholesterol and increased risk of cardiovascular disease. For all of these reasons, it is best to minimize your intake of high GI foods and maximize your intake of low GI foods. This book can show you how.

Research indicates that by choosing carbohydrates that are low GI as well as healthy (very important!), people may experience significant weight loss as well as decreased body fat, especially around the abdomen. By keeping blood sugar levels balanced, people also experience more even moods, reduced hunger cravings and increased metabolic rate—each an important factor in promoting long-term weight management and the prevention of chronic disease.

The glycemic index is a system of ranking all forms of carbohydrates (breads, rice, legumes, fruits and vegetables) on a scale of zero to one hundred according to how they impact the glycemic response. The glycemic response is how a carbohydrate affects blood glucose levels and consequently insulin levels (insulin is the hormone released by the pancreas to take glucose from the bloodstream and escort it to cells for energy utilization or storage as fat).

In the glycemic index scale, zero is the equivalent of water, which does not have any impact on blood glucose levels. And conversely, one hundred is the equivalent of pure glucose (sugar). If a food is digested quickly causing a rapid rise in blood glucose, hitting seventy or more on the glycemic index, it is cat-egorized as a high GI food. If a food is digested more slowly, causing a gradual release of blood glucose into the body, falling below fifty-five on the glycemic index, it is categorized as a low GI. Foods that fall between fifty-six and sixty-nine on the glycemic index are categorized as moderate GI foods.

High GI foods include bagels, soda crackers and french fries. High GI foods elicit a rapid conversion to blood glucose and, as a result, a dramatic insulin response. While high GI foods can be counted on to provide us with bursts of energy (what people often call a *sugar high* or *rush*), this energy is not sustain-able and most often is followed by an equally dramatic drop in energy (or *sugar low*) that may cause feelings of fatigue, sluggishness, slowed mental function, increased hunger and cravings, and sudden irritability. To counter these *sugar lows*, people crave and then consume more high GI foods, only to start the vicious bingeing-craving cycle all over again.

On the other side of the scale, low glycemic index foods such as plain yogurt, chick peas, crispy green lettuces and apples provide the body with sustained en-ergy, which reduces hunger and improves the manner in which the body utilizes energy reserves (stored as fat).

A New View on Carbohydrates

The term "glycemic index" was first coined by Professors David Jenkins and Tom Wolever from the Department of Nutritional Sciences, Faculty of Medicine, University of Toronto in Canada. Their research paper, "Glycemic Index of Foods: A Physiological Basis for Carbohydrate Exchange," was published in 1981 in the *American Journal of Clinical Nutrition* and revolutionized the way people un-derstood the role of carbohydrates in the diet. The researchers wanted to take an in-depth look at the food recommendations for diabetics. At that time it was believed that all simple carbohydrates caused a rapid rise in blood glucose levels and all complex carbohydrates released glucose more slowly into the body. Con-sequently, diabetics were advised to limit carbohydrate portions and eat more complex carbohyrdates to manage their blood sugar.

After the Canadian research was published however, a whole new view of carbohydrates emerged that challenged this previously held belief. Jenkins' and Wolever's results showed that the glycemic response of carbohydrates was not black and white; in fact, blood sugar responses varied considerably among various complex carbohydrates. The researchers concluded that certain carbohy-drates were better quality than others were. The biggest surprise was that certain starchy foods (such as white rice) were digested and absorbed more quickly than certain sugary foods. These results went against what was believed at the time. As a result, the research paper fueled a dramatic increase in curiosity, debate and ultimately clinical research on this topic all around the world. Thus, nutrition and medical experts, especially those working with people with diabetes, obesity and heart disease, needed to re-examine their recommendations for carbohydrate and sugar intake. Instead of only describing carbohydrates as complex or simple, now carbohydrates were also defined as low or high GI, and dietary recommendations were made accordingly.

How Is the Glycemic Index Measured?

To date, more than seven hundred foods have been classified according to their glycemic index (Foster-Powell et al. 2002). The GI value of a food is determined using scientific methods and cannot be calculated by simply analyzing the composition of a food. Currently, only a few nutrition research groups around the world provide a legitimate testing service. For over a decade, Professor Jennie Brand-Miller in the Human Nutrition Unit at the University of Sydney, Australia, co-author of *The New Glucose Revolution* and *The Low GI Diet Revolution*, has been at the forefront of glycemic index research. This research unit has measured the GI values of more than four hundred foods and counting. There is a GI value chart in Chapter five. For a more comprehensive list check out www.glycemicindex.com.

According to Brand-Miller and her collegues system, to measure a food's GI rating, a portion of a food containing fifty grams of carbohydrate is fed to ten healthy study participants, who fast overnight prior to the test. Blood samples are taken at fifteen to thirty minute intervals for two hours afterward. At a separate time, the same ten people eat an equal carbohydrate portion of glucose sugar (referred to as the control food) and again have their blood glucose responses measured for two hours. These two groups of blood samples are then tested and the blood glucose values are used to plot a graph or blood sugar response curve reflecting the two-hour period. The area under each curve (AUC) is calculated to reflect the total rise in blood glucose levels after eating the test and control foods. The GI rating is calculated by dividing the AUC for the test food by the AUC for the control food, and multiplying the result by one hundred. The average of the GI ratings from all ten participants is considered to be the official GI of that food.

Here are the reference ranges for the glycemic index:

Low GI = fifty-five or less
Moderate GI = fifty-six to sixty-nine
High GI = seventy or higher

Factors that Influence the Glycemic Index

GI values reflect the body's glucose response when that particular food is eaten and not combined with any other foods. GI values are also measured after a night of fasting. While that may be the case when we eat breakfast, it is not always so for lunch, dinner and snacks. So, we must understand that a variety of factors influence the glycemic index of a food including not only the aforementioned factors but also the type of starch, as well as the acid and sugar content. Dietary fibre, fat and protein content in a meal will cause carbohydrates to be digested more slowly, thus changing the overall glycemic impact of a meal. Finally, the cooking process is a factor; processed foods are digested more quickly while raw foods are digested more slowly. For example, raw carrots have a lower GI compared to cooked carrots. Cooking pasta *al dente* gives it a lower glycemic response compared to cooking it to a soft consistency.

What Is the Glycemic Load?

Now that you have a better understanding of the glycemic index, I'll introduce another term—the "glycemic load." The glycemic load takes us one step further than the glycemic index by providing a formula to calculate the "real life" impact of a carbohydrate in varying portion sizes. This formula was created by researchers at Harvard University in response to a limitation of the glycemic index. Specifically, since the the glycemic index is calculated based on a portion size that provides 50 grams of carbohydrate, it doesn't tell us the actual impact a typical portion will have on blood sugar. The glycemic load formula factors in a food's glycemic index value along with the grams of carbohydrate in a particular serving. For example, certain fruits and vegetables are moderate to high on the glycemic index (such as carrots, mango and watermelon) yet the amount of carbohydrate in a typical serving of these foods is low, thus they have a low glycemic load. To summarize, the glycemic load gives us the overall impact a food will have on blood sugar and insulin levels in different portion sizes.

Here is how the glycemic load is calculated:

Step 1: Start with the glycemic index rating of a single carbohydrate food and multiply that number by the amount (grams) of carbohydrate in the particular portion (this is available on label packaging).
Step 2: Take that resulting number and divide it by one hundred.

Here is an example:
The glycemic index for watermelon is seventy-two. There are six grams of carbohydrate in a one hundred and twenty gram serving. The glycemic load is $(72 \times 6) \div 100 = 4.3$

This is a perfect example of a food that has a high glycemic index but a low glycemic load because it contains a small amount of carbohydrates in a typical serving. Again, keep in mind, even if a food is moderate or high GI, if it contains very few carbohydrates per serving (such as watermelon, carrots and other fruits and vegetables), then the impact on blood sugar and insulin levels will not be great. If a food has both a high GI ranking and a high carbohydrate content (such as white bread and rice), it will have a high glycemic load and should be eaten in limited amounts.

The reference ranges for the glycemic load:

Low glycemic load = ten or less
Moderate glycemic load = eleven to nineteen
High glycemic load = twenty and higher

Low GI foods can be eaten in larger portions while high GI foods should be eaten in smaller portions to manage glycemic load. *That doesn't mean that you can eat low GI foods in unlimited amounts. It is important to keep the total glycemic load low at each meal.* When the total glycemic load of a meal is high, it triggers hormonal changes that promote fat storage. When the total glycemic load of a meal is low, it triggers your body to start actively using fat as an energy source.

In summary, despite the limitations of the glycemic index, it is still a good predictor of the impact carbohydrates have on blood sugar. In fact, a study published in the June 2006 issue of the *American Journal of Clinical Nutrition*, by researchers from the University of Toronto's Department of Nutritional Sciences, in partnership with top researchers at the University of Sydney, Australia, found that the GI was a reliable predictor of blood glucose whether the subjects consumed a single portion of one item or a normal meal. Even though the test meals varied in carbohydrate, fat and protein composition, the GI tables were ninety percent accurate in predicting the glucose response.

Use the glycemic index as an easy reference tool for your meal planning. If you want to know the impact of your particular serving size, use the glycemic load formula.

RESEARCH HIGHLIGHT:

In a 2006 study published in the *Archives of Internal Medicine*, researchers from the University of Sydney, Australia proved that low glycemic load diets reduce blood glucose and insulin levels. In this twelve-week controlled study, 129 overweight or obese people were randomly assigned one of four diets:

- High carbohydrate/low glycemic load
- High carbohydrate/high glycemic load
- High protein, carb reduced/ low glycemic load
- High protein, carb reduced/ high glycemic load

The participants were given calorie-restricted meal plans and access to a dietitian. Due to calorie-restrictions, all four diets resulted in weight loss of between four to six percent. However, the high carbohydrate/low glycemic index diet produced the best outcome, reducing both body fat and LDL (bad cholesterol). The diet that was high carbohydrate and high glycemic was associated with the slowest rate of weight loss. In the high carbohydrate diets, but not the high protein diet, lowering the glycemic load doubled the amount of body fat lost. The researchers concluded that even moderate reductions in glycemic load increase the rate of body fat loss, particularly for women. (*Archives of Internal Medicine* 2006; 166: 1466-1475).

INTERNATIONAL GI RESEARCH

Since the University of Toronto research paper was published in 1981, there has been a great deal of scientific study about the benefits of low GI foods. The studies have a common goal: they want to further understand the glycemic response and to document what benefits the varying responses might produce to prevent chronic diseases such as obesity, Type 2 diabetes, heart disease and cancer. Canada's University of Toronto and Australia's University of Sydney are leading research hubs on the glycemic index, but there are also ongoing studies around the world. Here is a sampling of compelling published research to date:

- In a 1999 issue of *Pediatrics*, a group of researchers from Tufts University in Boston reported a relationship between a high glycemic diet, overeating and obesity. They evaluated the food intake of twelve obese teenage boys after three separate meals (low GI, moderate GI and high GI), and found that the boys consumed significantly more food after a moderate GI and high GI meal than after a low GI meal. The researchers concluded, *"The rapid absorption of glucose after consumption of high GI meals induces a sequence of hormonal and metabolic changes that promote excessive food intake in obese subjects."*
- Research published in *Diabetes Care* in 2000 found that high blood glucose levels or repeated glycemic "spikes" following a meal may promote Type 2 diabetes and coronary heart disease by increasing oxidative damage to the cardiovascular system and also by directly increasing insulin levels.
- In 2002, the University of Toronto partnered with researchers in France and Sweden in an overview published in the *American Journal of Clinical Nutrition*. They said, *"The glycemic index has particular relevance to those chronic Western diseases associated with central obesity and insulin resistance."*
- Also in 2002, published in the *European Journal of Clinical Nutrition*, a group of researchers from Toronto, France and Italy looked at the scientific evidence and role of the glycemic index on chronic Western disease. They found several health benefits exist for reducing the rate of carbohydrate absorption by means of a low GI diet, including, reduced insulin demand, improved blood glucose control and reduced blood lipid levels.
- In 2004, a study published in the *American Journal of Clinical Nutrition* found that lowering the GI of food intake could yield the same effects on glucose response as being on a low-carb diet.
- In 2004, a study revealed that high insulin levels, or a high sugar diet (which causes high insulin levels), are connected with a higher incidence of prostate cancer. (*Journal of Cancer* 2004;112:446). It was shown in a previous study that increased insulin levels are associated with more advanced prostate cancer (*British Journal of Cancer* 2002; 87: 726).
- In 2004, a prospective study by Canadian researchers in the *International Journal of Cancer* (2005; 114(4): 653-658) found that post-menopausal women with

high overall dietary glycemic index values were at increased risk of breast cancer. A prospective study in the United States found that premenopausal women with high overall dietary glycemic index values and low levels of physical activity were also at increased risk of breast cancer (*Cancer Epidemiology Biomarkers & Prevention* 2004;13(1):65-70).

- According to articles in the *Journal of the National Cancer Institute* (2002; 94:1293-1300 and 2004;96(3):229-233) there are some studies that suggest increased risk of colorectal cancer with a high glycemic diet.

- In 2005, the *American Journal of Clinical Nutrition* published a report that said people lost more weight on a "slow carb" or low-glycemic-load diet than on a low-fat or low-carb diet. After twelve months on the various diets, the slow-carb group lost 7.8 percent of their body weight compared with 6.1 percent in the low-fat-diet group. The levels of triglycerides (blood fats linked to heart disease) were also decreased by thirty-seven percent in the slow-carb group versus nineteen percent in the low-fat group.

For more information on current clinical studies, visit www.glycemicindex.com. This is the "Home of the Glycemic Index," run by the Human Nutrition Unit, School of Molecular and Microbial Biosciences at the University of Sydney and top glycemic index expert Professor Jennie Brand-Miller. Each month, the site offers a free e-newsletter with research updates as well as lifestyle and diet tips. This is a terrific resource to stay informed on glycemic index research.

The Glycemic Research Institute in Washington DC, on the web at www. glycemic.com, is also another valuable resource for up-to-date clinical data.

So, Is the GI the Next "IT" Diet?

Don't misinterpret the hype surrounding the glycemic index. Although following a low GI diet can help promote weight loss, the GI is not intended or promoted as a weight-loss tool unto itself. You will achieve the best results if you combine a low GI diet with regular exercise, adequate sleep, stress management and smart supplements.

Following a low GI diet is not a fad; this is a new way of eating that is here to stay and that's what makes it so important. It's a revolutionary way of understanding and choosing foods. And here's why...this sensible approach to eating is metabolism-driven, promotes satiety (satisfaction from meals), allows for variances in the diet and has significant, well-documented benefits for overall health.

The chart of low/moderate/high GI carbohydrate values (which appears on page 51 of this book) offers you a guide when choosing which carbohydrates to consume. Eating low GI foods is healthy, nutritious and easy to follow. This is particularly important because most fad diets, such as the low-carb or no-carb diets are difficult to sustain in the long-term, and can be detrimental to your health. The GI offers an alternative that allows the intake of carbohydrates, but promotes the consumption of low GI carbohydrates such as fruits, vegetables, whole grains, legumes and nuts—these are the healthy, high-fibre carbohydrates. More importantly, the GI offers significant benefits for blood sugar control and lowering the risk of chronic disease.

THE HEALTH BENEFITS OF EATING LOW GI FOODS

The health benefits of a low GI diet are widespread and well documented. They include improved weight control, enhanced blood sugar management, and most importantly, decreased risk of diabetes, high cholesterol and heart disease. Overtime, a low GI diet can promote fat loss, especially around the abdomen, and modify appetite and food cravings to a more normal level. Digestion and bowel function can improve, since eating more vegetables, fruit and other quality sources of soluble fibre can lessen constipation and diarrhea. Finally, there are secondary benefits from balanced blood sugar, such as improved sleep patterns, improved skin condition and increased vitality.

All of the benefits from a low GI diet begin and end with enhanced blood sugar and insulin management. Let's take a closer look at this topic to better understand the role of insulin in your health.

3
CHAPTER
The Role of Insulin

Insulin is often thought of only in its relationship to people with diabetes. Yet, insulin plays a critical role in the functioning of everyone's body. Furthermore, insulin is one of the few hormones involved in fat storage, so for those people trying to lose weight, understanding the role of insulin must be part of the weight-loss equation.

When we eat carbohydrates, they are broken down into glucose, which causes a rise in blood sugar. Insulin is the hormone secreted by the pancreas in response to that rise in blood sugar. Insulin's role is to transport the excess blood sugar from the blood stream and facilitate its transition into cells throughout the body to be utilized as energy. Thus, insulin helps return blood sugar levels to normal. Insulin also aids in the production of enzymes, hormones and muscles.

UNDERSTANDING INSULIN RESISTANCE

When blood sugar levels are balanced, the body functions as it should. This meaning blood sugar levels rise modestly after a meal, insulin is released to bring blood sugar into the cells to be used for energy, and then blood sugar levels return to normal. However, if we eat too many refined, high glycemic carbohydrates, and continually have high blood sugar, then increasing amounts of insulin are released. If insulin levels are chronically elevated, then the cells of your body eventually become resistant to the action of insulin. This is called insulin resistance. Once insulin resistance occurs, insulin becomes ineffective in its job to move glucose into the cells to be burned for energy, so blood glucose levels remain high. In response, the pancreas releases more insulin to try and reduce blood glucose levels. The end result is high, uncontrolled blood glucose *and* high insulin levels. It is estimated that over twenty-five percent of the population suffers with high blood glucose levels and insulin resistance.

Aside from eating a high GI diet, other factors that increase the risk of insulin resistance include the following:

- Genetics—inherited defects with insulin receptors
- Inactivity—a sedentary lifestyle
- Obesity—body fat releases a hormone called resistin that reduces insulin sensitivity

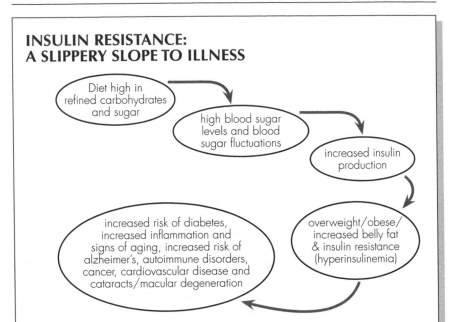

INSULIN RESISTANCE: A SLIPPERY SLOPE TO ILLNESS

Diet high in refined carbohydrates and sugar

high blood sugar levels and blood sugar fluctuations

increased insulin production

overweight/obese/ increased belly fat & insulin resistance (hyperinsulinemia)

increased risk of diabetes, increased inflammation and signs of aging, increased risk of alzheimer's, autoimmune disorders, cancer, cardiovascular disease and cataracts/macular degeneration

Poor blood sugar regulation is the first step towards insulin resistance. Insulin resistance is a pre-diabetic condition that increases the risk of obesity, cardiovascular disease, kidney disease, nerve problems, and polycystic ovary disease. Insulin resistance occurs when the body becomes resistant or "*immune*" to the action of its own insulin (which normally pushes glucose into cells) and requires more insulin to do the same job, flooding the body with insulin and causing serious secondary repercussions.

DIABETES BREAKDOWN

Diabetes is a chronic disease in which the pancreas produces insufficient amounts of insulin or the body does not respond appropriately to the insulin produced (insulin resistance). There are two main forms of diabetes: Type 1 (formerly known as juvenile-onset diabetes or insulin-dependent diabetes) and Type 2 (formerly known as adult-onset diabetes or non-insulin dependent diabetes).

Type 1 diabetes is often called juvenile diabetes because it primarily occurs in children or adolescents. This form accounts for only about ten percent of diabetes cases. In Type 1 diabetes, the cells that produce insulin (beta cells) become damaged or are destroyed. In infants and children, beta cells are usually destroyed rapidly, causing a sudden rise in blood sugar levels. In adults, they are destroyed more slowly, causing a slower rise in blood sugar levels. Typically, people with Type 1 diabetes need to have insulin injections to ensure their blood sugar levels in the bloodstream do not exceed dangerous levels. (Remember, insulin transports blood sugar out of the bloodstream and into cells.)

The exact cause of Type 1 diabetes is unknown, but it is thought that the immune system attacks and destroys the beta cells. Those with a family history face a greater risk of contracting the disease. There is no cure for type 1 diabetes however lifestyle measures (exercise and diet) and supplements are helpful in improving blood sugar regulation and increasing insulin sensitivity. If you suffer from Type 1 diabetes, work with your healthcare provider or naturopathic doctor to find out complementary ways to support your condition.

INTERNATIONAL DIABETES STATISTICS

In 1998, the World Health Organization published a report that estimated the number of people with diabetes was 135 million worldwide. However, less than a decade later, that estimate jumped to 194 million. According to the International Diabetes Federation, diabetes now affects more than 230 million people worldwide and is expected to affect 350 million by 2025. Diabetes is the fourth or fifth leading cause of death in developed countries, and is responsible for over one million amputations each year. In 2003, the five countries with the largest numbers of people with diabetes were India (35.5 million), China (23.8 million), the United States (16 million), Russia (9.7 million) and Japan (6.7 million). By 2025, the number of people with diabetes is expected to more than double in Africa, the Eastern Mediterranean and Middle East and Southeast Asia. The incidence of diabetes is expected to rise by 20 percent in Europe, 50 percent in North America, 85 percent in South and Central America, and 75 percent in the Western Pacific.

Type 2 diabetes accounts for the remaining ninety percent of diabetes cases. In the past, this form was called adult-onset diabetes but the greatest increase of Type 2 diabetes in recent years has occurred among children and adolescents. Type 2 diabetes occurs when the body stops producing enough insulin or, as is more often the case, the body becomes resistant to the insulin that is produced and as a result glucose cannot enter the cells to be used as energy and so blood sugar levels remain elevated.

When blood sugar levels are high the pancreas produces more insulin than usual to try to compensate for the body's inefficiency, a condition known as hyperinsulinemia (high insulin). Gradually, insulin secretion from the pancreas falters, and eventually stops, leading to full-blown diabetes.

This scenario doesn't happen overnight. Studies have suggested that insulin resistance develops many years before the onset of Type 2 diabetes—so there is a long period of "warning." Initially there aren't any symptoms of insulin resistance, and it can only be determined by laboratory tests (fasting blood sugar and a glucose tolerance test). The majority of people who have insulin resistance eventually develop Type 2 diabetes and metabolic syndrome. Type 2 diabetes is often accompanied by symptoms of mood swings, irritability, hunger, thirst and sometimes food cravings may occur.

Risk factors associated with Type 2 diabetes include a genetic predisposition, poor diet (high sugar, high glycemic), sedentary lifestyle (inactive), being overweight or obese, ethnicity (Black, Hispanic, and Native American) and environmental factors. Type 2 diabetes is also more common among those over age forty-five, however it is not truly an age-related disease. The incidence increases with age because people tend to exercise less, lose muscle mass and gain weight as they age. Today, diabetes is also having a dramatic impact among children and adolescents due to poor diets, lack of activity and the rise in obesity among younger people.

The link between obesity, insulin resistance and Type 2 diabetes is very strong. Over eighty percent of people with Type 2 diabetes are overweight or obese and ninety-two percent of people with Type 2 diabetes have insulin resistance. Researchers now refer to these coexisting conditions as "*diabesity*".

BLOOD SUGAR HIGHS AND LOWS

Since insulin is critical in the processing of glucose into usable energy, a lack of it results in increased blood glucose levels and a condition known as hyperglycemia. Hyperglycemia is an excess of blood sugar in the body. It results in frequent and excessive thirst, hunger and urination. Other symptoms may include dry mouth, itchy skin, fatigue and recurrent infections. Hypoglycemia, on the other hand, occurs when blood sugar levels drop under normal levels causing dizziness and the shakes, sudden sweating and nausea, racing heart and general mental confusion. The symptoms may be temporary until blood sugar levels are restored. Hypoglycemia may occur for those with diabetes, but may also be triggered by poor diet and lifestyle. Both hyper- and hypoglycemia may be precursors to diabetes and can have serious, even fatal consequences, if left untreated. If you suffer the symptoms of either condition, consult with your healthcare provider immediately to determine the root cause, and to address diet and lifestyle factors.

INSULIN AND METABOLIC SYNDROME

Metabolic syndrome is a term given to a collection of symptoms that increase one's risk of heart disease, stroke and diabetes. Metabolic syndrome was formerly called Syndrome X and is marked by insulin resistance, elevated levels of cholesterol and triglycerides and abdominal obesity. Each of these factors alone is dangerous to health, but having them together greatly increases the risk of developing chronic disease.

Metabolic Syndrome is diagnosed when a person has three or more of the following characteristics:

- Abdominal obesity—waist circumference greater than 102 cm (40 inches) in men, and 88 cm (35 inches) in women
- High triglyceride levels—above 150 mg/dL

- Low HDL cholesterol levels—less than 40 mg/dL in men and 50 mg/dL in women
- High blood pressure—greater than or equal to 130/85 mm Hg
- Insulin resistance
- High fasting glucose level—with fasting blood sugar (more than 110 mg/dL)

The underlying cause of metabolic syndrome is insulin resistance. It is the key factor to creating the metabolic changes that lead to weight gain, elevated cholesterol, high blood pressure and then eventually Type 2 diabetes and heart disease.

Some experts estimate that as many as one in four, or forty-seven million adults in the United States, have metabolic syndrome. These numbers are expected to rise as the population ages. Keep in mind that age is not the cause of metabolic syndrome. The key risk factors for developing this condition—inactivity and obesity—are simply more prevalent in older adults. In fact, approximately forty percent of those over age sixty have metabolic syndrome.

INSULIN AND APPETITE: WHAT'S THE CONNECTION?

Insulin has widespread influence on the body, and can even increase appetite. Studies show that regular consumption of high glycemic meals results in insulin "spikes" and subsequent low blood sugar, triggering hunger and food cravings for more high glycemic foods. High glycemic foods, like bagels, white rice or donuts, are broken down into sugar very quickly creating a strong insulin response and exposing your body to the harmful effects of high insulin. While eating high glycemic foods provides bursts of energy, this is generally followed by hunger, fatigue, restlessness, severe mood swings and depleted energy, which leads to further bingeing and craving cycles. So the energy burst is temporary and followed by a crash, which sends us snacking on more high glycemic foods.

Conversely, low GI foods are digested and absorbed more slowly through the intestine, which naturally promotes satiety or the feeling of satisfaction from a meal. Foods that are low GI make you feel fuller longer while foods that are high GI may increase appetite and hunger.

Low glycemic index foods like fruits and vegetables provide a sustained release of energy, which reduces hunger and facilitates burning fat for energy. Because they slow the release of glucose into the bloodstream, they promote better insulin control. Plus these foods provide rich sources of vitamins, minerals and fiber—essential nutrients for good health.

SUGAR: NOT SO SWEET

Do you crave comfort foods such as soda pop, chocolate, candy, or cookies on a daily basis? If so, you're not alone. Sweets are a weakness for many of us. In fact, the average person consumes 160 pounds of sugar each year. It's true. Four cans of cola daily, each can providing thirty-nine grams (1.375 ounces) of sugar, would

---

CAN YOU EAT TOO MANY LOW GI FOODS?

Yes. A low GI ranking does not mean that food can be eaten in unlimited amounts. Common sense must still prevail. Certain diet programs rank foods and theorize that the lower the ranking, the more of that particular food may be consumed. This is misleading because excess calories—taking in more than you expend in energy—can be stored as fat, regardless of whether those calories come from carbohydrates, protein or fat. Remember that the GI is only a guide to understand the body's blood glucose response to various forms of carbohydrates. You must still exercise portion control.

Studies show that people who regularly eat large portions not only have a higher tendency to struggle with weight issues, but also have an increased risk of chronic disease and shortened lifespan. Small portions, on the other hand, have been linked to a healthier lifestyle and greater longevity.

This being said, however, there are certain low GI foods, such as nutrient- and fiber-rich vegetables and non-tropical fruit that can be eaten in larger portions.

---

alone account for 125 pounds of sugar per year. The obvious sources of sugar are candy, cookies and other baked goods, but most of us don't think about the hidden sources, such as ketchup, salad dressing, peanut butter, snack bars and mayonnaise. All these add up to too much sugar, and potential health risks.

Numerous studies have shown that a diet high in refined sugar has been linked to diabetes, obesity, elevated triglycerides (a type of blood fat), tooth decay, poor immune function and allergies. Plus high-sugar foods are high in the glycemic index, and we know what that can do to us.

Sugar or sweet cravings are often driven by imbalances in blood sugar levels. When blood sugar is low, which occurs an hour or so after a high GI meal, we crave more sweets. The body gets used to, and begins to depend on, a regular supply of refined sugar. Even though the body does not respond well to high blood sugar levels, it also naturally seeks balance and therefore wants its energy supply, and subsequent bodily function such as hormone production, to remain constant. Overindulging in sweets can affect both physical and emotional well-being, causing headaches, fatigue, mood swings, irritability, anxiety and impaired mental function.

INSULIN AND BODY FAT: WHAT'S THE CONNECTION?

Insulin resistance and body fat share a reciprocal and rather unhealthy relationship. High insulin levels cause us to store more fat, and carrying excess fat reduces insulin sensitivity and increases the risk of insulin resistance. Sound confusing? Let me explain further.

Insulin is intimately connected to our potential for fat burning and fat storage. High insulin levels reduce the levels of lipoprotein lipase, the enzyme which releases fat from storage to be used as energy. As a result, more fat is stored

A SWEET ALTERNATIVE

For better health, avoid refined sugar. If you crave something sweet, have a piece of low GI fruit such as an apple or other non-tropical fruit. Dried fruits provide concentrated sources of vitamins and minerals along with fibre, but are moderate to high GI so consume in moderation and watch your portion size. Good food sweeteners to consider are honey, maple syrup, malt syrups and date sugar. These products provide some nutritional value and are not as hard on blood sugar levels as refined sugar. In baked goods, mashed bananas and apples are a great substitute for sugar. Artificial sweeteners such as aspartame and saccharin should be avoided because they have been linked to health concerns. Stevia, a sweetener obtained from a plant in Latin America, appears to be a safe sugar substitute. Depending on how it is processed, Stevia can provide up to 300 times the sweetening power of sugar—without the calories. (Quality stevia products are available at health food stores.)

because that enzyme is reduced. On the other hand, low insulin levels increase levels of a hormone called glucagon, which allows fat to be burned for energy. As long as insulin levels remain high, fat remains in storage and the body will continue to use glucose for its energy needs.

APPLES VERSUS PEARS: WHERE IS YOUR FAT?

Researchers have discovered that it's not just how much extra body fat a person carries, but where the fat is stored on the body that increases their risk of disease. People who tend to store excess fat around their middle, nicknamed apples, are more likely to develop serious health problems (such as Type 2 diabetes, high cholesterol and blood pressure, coronary heart disease and stroke) than people who store their excess fat in their hips and thighs, nicknamed pears. An apple-shaped body is characterized by a potbelly or spare tire. This abdominal or "visceral fat" indicates that there is excess fat surrounding the internal organs. Excess belly fat is also an indicator of a condition called *metabolic syndrome*. Other signs of metabolic syndrome include elevated blood pressure, high triglycerides, insulin resistance and low levels of HDL cholesterol (the "good" cholesterol)—factors which also increase the risk of diabetes and heart disease.

KNOW YOUR RISK

A waist circumference of more than forty inches for men or more than thirty-five inches for women is associated with a substantially increased risk of developing disease.

Abdominal obesity is influenced by a number of factors including genetics and lifestyle choices. Doing physical activity, not smoking and using unsaturated fat over saturated fat have been shown to decrease the risk of developing abdominal obesity.

Source: C. Gasteyger and A. Tremblay "Metabolic Impact of Body Fat Distribution," *Journal of Endocrinological Investigation* 2002;25: 876-883.

BELLY FAT IS A WARNING SIGN OF THINGS TO COME

We know now that belly fat greatly increases your chance of developing insulin resistance and diabetes.

- According to a study presented at The First Annual World Congress on the Insulin Resistance Syndrome, Los Angeles, California (November 2003), at a body mass index of greater than twenty-five, sixty percent of individuals had insulin resistance; and at a waist circumference greater than 88 centimetres in women or 102 centimetres in men, sixty-eight percent had insulin resistance.
- In a study published in *Diabetes Care* in 2006, researchers measured insulin resistance and compared it to several risk factors for diabetes in men and women including heart-lung fitness, whole body fatness and abdominal obesity. The results revealed that while a lack of physical fitness and being overweight were significant predictors of diabetes in men and women, the primary predictor of insulin resistance, the precursor to Type 2 diabetes, is storing fat in the belly rather than the hips.

To burn fat for energy and reduce belly fat, blood sugar levels must be balanced and insulin levels must be lowered. And, this can be achieved through proper diet, nutritional supplements and exercise, outlined in the coming chapters.

INSULIN AND STRESS: WHAT'S THE CONNECTION?

Cortisol is a hormone released from the adrenal glands in response to stress or those "fight or flight" situations (rush hour traffic, deadlines). Approximately half of all adults suffer the adverse effects of stress, such as muscle tension, high blood pressure, insomnia and depression. Most recently, stress has been linked to obesity. When a person experiences chronic stress, cortisol levels rise. This causes the body to store more fat around the belly, which reduces insulin sensitivity.

The news on cortisol is not all bad. Cortisol is the most important hormone for blood sugar and insulin regulation. In response to a stressful event, cortisol helps your body become more effective at producing glucose from protein, a process called gluconeogenesis, so that it can accommodate the increased energy requirements. This protein comes from existing body structures, such as muscle, skin, and organs. If this happens occasionally and is short term, there is not a problem, however when stress is chronic, this process can lead to muscle loss (wasting)—another factor that can contribute to weight gain because loss of muscle means that metabolism is reduced.

During stress, cortisol reduces insulin sensitivity and the utilization of glucose for energy so that there is increased blood sugar available to be used by the central nervous system or your brain. Your brain is the only organ in the body that can absorb glucose directly, without the action of insulin. Your brain uses approximately one hundred grams of glucose daily, and during times of high stress, it demands even more. Cortisol functions to increase the amount of glucose available in your body in order to accommodate the brain's increased desire for glucose. Researchers believe that insulin resistance often develops in part as a coping mechanism to feed the brain with necessary glucose.

The release of cortisol in response to stress was designed to help the body quickly increase energy supplies to meet the immediate demands, however because chronic stress levels associated with Western lifestyles keep us in this "fight or flight" mode continuously, the risk of developing full-blown insulin resistance increases (from a prolonged decrease in insulin sensitivity) and weight gain occurs (remember excess insulin increases fat storage).

Stress isn't the only factor that raises cortisol. Eating too many sweet, simple carbohydrates can also elevate cortisol levels. When you eat a high GI food, such as a candy bar, the body generates a strong insulin response, to bring blood sugar down. This strong insulin response can trigger a dramatic drop in blood sugar for three to five hours after the snack. When blood glucose levels fall, this triggers a surge of adrenaline and cortisol. This can result in anxiety, irritability, nervousness and palpitations. A classic example of this is how children behave when they have eaten too much sugar. Continual consumption of high GI, sugary foods can lead to fluctuations of insulin, glucose and adrenal hormones throughout the day, with consequences on both physical and emotional well-being.

INSULIN AND AGING: WHAT'S THE CONNECTION?

Poorly regulated blood sugar and insulin levels are major contributors to accelerated aging. As production and effectiveness of insulin falters, glucose builds up in the blood stream causing a series of health problems that many people associate with normal aging. For example, we have all heard the expression about the mid-life spread. Gaining fat around the abdomen is a consequence of uncontrolled blood sugar, insulin resistance, stress, and lack of activity—lifestyle factors. Because these factors affect us more as we age, people mistakenly think they are a result of aging, when in reality they are a sign of an underlying hormonal imbalance.

Elevated blood sugar leads to the formation of advanced glycation endproducts, also known as AGE. Excess blood sugar binds to proteins found in skin, cartilage, muscle, blood vessels and other tissues causing wrinkling, stiffening and malfunctioning, leading to accelerated aging. When blood vessels and nerves become stiff and hardened (glycated) blood flow to the organs and extremities is impaired. In the extremities this can be noticed as "pins and needles" or numbness in the hands and feet. Poor circulation to the blood vessels in the pelvic area can result in erectile dysfunction, which is a common consequence of uncontrolled diabetes and high blood sugar.

If hemoglobin (the oxygen-binding protein in red blood cells) is encrusted with glucose, the brain, heart and muscles receive less oxygen causing all functions to decrease. This results in lack of energy and premature aging.

Connective tissue (collagen) is also affected by excess sugar resulting in skin wrinkles. Cataracts may develop as a result to damage to the lens of the eye, which is made of protein. If the same problem affects the retina, blindness may be the result. Mental acuity may also be affected.

Insulin also activates genes that produce a number of mediators of inflammation, so with high insulin, the level of inflammation in your body increases. The joints become swollen and inflexible as the symptoms of arthritis set in.

High blood sugar and elevated insulin may increase your risk of degenerative brain diseases such as dementia and Alzheimer's disease. But that's not all—high blood glucose levels affect the function of many proteins and enzymes, such that the chances of dying prematurely from any cause are higher. You don't need to be in the diabetic range to be at risk. High glucose and insulin levels fuel the growth of abnormal cells that cause various types of cancer including, breast, colon, endometrial and pancreatic.

INSULIN AND HEART DISEASE: WHAT'S THE CONNECTION?

Heart disease claims more lives every year than any other affliction, and is particularly worrisome for diabetics. According to the American Heart Association (AHA), sixty-three percent of people with diabetes experience symptoms of cardiovascular disease. In fact, the AHA estimates that three-quarters of people with diabetes will die of some form of heart or blood vessel disease.

It is not just diabetics that need to be worried about heart disease. Those with pre-diabetes, those who eat high glycemic diets and those with insulin resistance are also at increased risk of heart disease for a variety of reasons. High glycemic diets can lead to hyperinsulinemia and insulin resistance, which can lead to obesity, hypertension, hyperlipidemia (elevated cholesterol), and diabetes, all major risk factors for heart disease. As well, a study published in the *American Journal of Clinical Nutrition* in 2002 reported a significant association between diets with a high glycemic load and increased levels of C-reactive protein (a protein indicator of inflammation and a distinct marker for disease, particularly heart disease).

Another risk factor for heart disease, hypertension, often results secondary to being obese. Excess body weight increases the workload and stress to the heart, which leads to hypertension. When insulin levels are high the body retains sodium, which also increases blood pressure.

The connection between insulin and cholesterol is a little more complicated. High insulin levels trigger the release of free fatty acids into the bloodstream. The liver responds by increasing triglycerides, and this increases high density lipoprotein (HDL) excretion from the body, lowering your blood HDL (good) cholesterol levels. These changes also cause the LDL (bad) cholesterol to become smaller and more dense, which makes it more likely to form as plaque on the inside of blood vessels. So, to summarize, the net result of high insulin is elevated triglycerides, low HDL cholesterol, and an increase in small dense LDL cholesterol: a combination of factors known to substantially increase the risk of cardiovascular disease.

The good news is that studies show that following a diet of low GI foods improves insulin response and can reduce risk factors for heart disease. Specifically, a low GI diet has been shown to increase levels of HDL (good cholesterol) and decrease levels of LDL (bad cholesterol). Several reports also indicate that low glycemic diets are associated with lower triglycerides levels (another marker for heart disease). One study published in the *Current Atherosclerosis Reports* (Nov. 3, 2001) found that substituting low GI for high GI foods can lower triglycerides by fifteen to twenty-five percent. A low GI diet can also help facilitate weight loss, which in turn helps reduce two other risk factors for heart disease: blood pressure and cholesterol.

HEART DISEASE WAKE-UP CALL!

According to the Center for Disease Control in the US, cardiovascular disease (CVD) is the leading cause of death in men and women in Canada, the US, China, Europe and Australia. Heart attack and stroke are responsible for twice as many deaths in women in the US, than from all forms of cancer combined. Both the World Heart Organization and the World Health Organization report that CVD kills up to seventeen million people each year. In developing countries, CVD is on the rise, afflicting people at an earlier age than in developed nations. Up to eighty percent of the world's deaths by CVD are now reported in developing or middle-income nations. By 2020, CVD will be the leading cause of death worldwide (with the exception of sub-Saharan Africa), surpassing communicable diseases. However, there is hope. National education efforts and individual action can reduce the risk of disability or death from CVD by up to fifty percent. The leading risk factors for CVD include, in order, hypertension, high blood cholesterol, diabetes, obesity, cigarette smoking and inactivity. These are what we call *modifiable* risk factors because we have control over them.

4

CHAPTER

Make the Most Out of Your Macronutrients

If you're going to follow the glycemic index, choosing to eat mostly low or moderate GI carbohydrates, you still need to make healthy choices in the other facets of your diet, namely protein and fat intake. These food groups provide us with necessary nutrients for health. In addition, protein and fat eaten with carbohydrates slows digestion and lowers the glycemic impact of a meal. In fact, there has been speculation that the low-fat craze of the 1980s may be partially responsible for the increase in the instances of blood sugar problems, insulin resistance and diabetes. This is because when fat was taken out of foods, often substituted with increased starch and sugar, the foods became higher GI foods.

So, in order to take what we've learned about the glycemic index and put it into action, as outlined in the next chapter, we first need to understand the key components of a healthy diet—the macronutrients.

Macronutrients consist of carbohydrates, proteins and fats. They are called "macro" because we need these nutrients in large quantities, compared to the micronutrients (vitamins and minerals), which are needed in smaller quantities. Our bodies need a balance of quality protein, carbohydrates and fats in order to function at their best. These macronutrients provide us with the energy and nutrients needed for proper growth, development, and many body processes. Striking the right balance of macronutrients is key for health and weight management.

RECOMMENDED MACRONUTRIENT INTAKE

The Institute of Medicine recommends ranges for macronutrient intake that are associated with a reduced risk of chronic disease while providing adequate intake of essential nutrients. They suggest adults get forty-five to sixty-five percent of their calories from carbohydrates, twenty to thirty-five percent from fat, and ten to thirty-five percent from protein. Ranges for children are similar, except that infants and younger children need a slightly higher proportion of fat (twenty-five to forty percent).

CARBOHYDRATES

We have discussed carbohydrates and their relationship to blood sugar and insulin, but there is more to know about this heavily scrutinized food group.

Carbohydrates are the body's main source of fuel—glucose—that is needed by every cell in our body. They also provide valuable nutrients (vitamins, minerals and essential fatty acids) and fiber, which is important for intestinal health, weight management and blood sugar balance.

CARBOHYDRATE FOOD SOURCES

Carbohydrates are typically classified as either simple or complex. Simple carbohydrates include naturally occurring sugars in milk and fruit, and refined sugars (granulated sugar). There are some major differences among these carbohydrates: fruits offer a range of nutrients and fiber, and are typically low to moderate GI, while refined sugars provide "empty calories" (lack nutritional value) and are high GI. As noted earlier, excess sugar consumption is associated with numerous health problems. The World Health Organization recommends reducing sugar intake to below ten percent of total calories. Aside from candy and baked goods, sugar is also found in pop, condiments (ketchup, barbecue sauce), juices, ice cream and other sweets. These are the foods that you want to limit as they are high on the glycemic index as well as loaded with empty calories.

Complex carbohydrates include starches and indigestible dietary fiber. Starches are found in bread, pasta, rice, beans and some vegetables. Today many of our starches are refined and processed which strips the food of its fiber and nutrients, and as a result increases its GI. For example, white bread, pasta and rice are much less nutritious and have high GIs, so choose the brown or whole grain versions.

Dietary fiber is found in fruits, vegetables, beans and the indigestible parts of whole-grains such as wheat and oat bran. In addition to supporting intestinal health and proper elimination, fiber also improves blood sugar balance (reduces a food's GI), lowers cholesterol, reduces the risk of colon and breast cancer, and plays a role in weight management.

EAT YOUR ROUGHAGE

There are two types of dietary fiber: insoluble and soluble. Both forms are found in most foods, but in varying amounts.

Foods that contain insoluble fiber include beans and lentils, brown rice, fruits with edible seeds, oats, and wheat bran. Insoluble fiber has a bulking effect in the stomach, which slows digestion and absorption. It also improves elimination (and relieves constipation) by absorbing water, and swelling within the intestine, which helps pull and remove waste materials from the body. Choose whole-grain breads and cereals over refined products as the refining process strips away most of the fiber and nutrients.

Soluble fiber can be found in all fruit and vegetables including, legumes, green vegetables, potatoes, apples and strawberries. Soluble fiber mixes with water in a meal to form a gel in the stomach, which traps waste and helps lower LDL (bad) cholesterol.

The recommended intake of fiber for adults fifty years and younger is thirty-eight grams for men and twenty-five grams for women; for men and women over fifty the recommended intake is thirty and twenty-one grams per day, respectively, due to decreased food consumption. Sadly, most people get only around one-third of the recommended amount. To boost fiber intake, incorporate more raw vegetables, fruits, whole-grains and legumes in your diet and consider a fiber supplement.

THE LOWDOWN OF LOW CARBOHYDRATE DIETS

Low carb diets are based on the scientific premise that without sufficient glucose for energy, the body will turn to its fat stores to burn for energy. As such, in the short-term at least, low carb diets help encourage weight loss. However, low carb diets raise some potential long-term problems. The first problem is that people tend not to be able to maintain a low carb diet. Once they start eating carbohydrates again, they tend to regain the weight they lost. This frustration may lead to yo-yo or more drastic forms of dieting.

THE CARBOHYDRATE CONUNDRUM SOLVED

Complex carbohydrates are a healthy choice for your diet—high fiber whole-grains (whole wheat, brown rice, oats and flaxseed), along with legumes, beans and vegetables. High fiber foods are broken down more slowly and evenly, which helps to control blood sugar levels. These foods also play a role in reducing cholesterol levels and reducing your risk of cancer. Processed foods, containing refined sugars and flours, and foods high in starch, are broken down more quickly, resulting in undesirable short, high bursts in blood sugar levels. These are high GI foods, and should be minimized.

The GI of a food is influenced by several factors: the amount of carbohydrates it contains, the types of sugar found in it (glucose, lactose, sucrose), the type and quantity of starch and the way it is cooked. Some ingredients (e.g. fats, tannins and lectins) can decrease a food's GI because they slow the digestion process. However, the factor that most affects the GI is the amount of carbohydrates a food contains.

In 2002, the National Institutes of Health (NIH) advised that a range of carbohydrate intakes could adequately meet the body's needs while minimizing the risk of disease. They recommended carbs comprise forty-five to sixty-five percent of energy, while fat (twenty-five to thirty-five percent of energy) and protein (fifteen to thirty-five percent of energy) comprise the rest. The American Heart Association has reported that people can restrict carbs to only forty percent of energy without posing any danger to their health. The Canadian Diabetes Association recommends that diabetics count carbohydrates and try to consume roughly the same amount of carbohydrates from meal to meal, and day to day.

The second problem is that low carb diets also deprive the cells of their primary energy source (glucose). When this happens, the body uses glycogen stored in the liver and converts it into glucose. Once glycogen is depleted, the body converts fat and protein into glucose for a source of fuel. The use of protein, which comes from muscle, can result in muscle wasting. When fat is used to provide energy, the liver takes fatty acids and produces compounds called ketone bodies. This is known as ketosis. Some consider ketosis to be a sign of dieting success. However, if the brain is utilizing ketones for energy (instead of proper glucose) then it is not working at its best and mental function may decrease (i.e. sluggish, scattered brain, impaired judgement and impaired memory). The brain is the most energy-intensive organ in the body, responsible for over half our energy requirements. The benefits of carbs on mental performance are well documented. Long-term low carb dieting can impair brain and nervous system function.

Lastly, low carb diets often result in deficiencies of vitamins, minerals and essential fatty acids, because these nutrients are obtained from eating vegetables, fruits and whole-grains—which are restricted on a low carb diet.

Due to the concerns that came about from the low carb diets, and the necessity of carbohydrates for brain function, the Institute of Medicine made a recommendation that adults consume a minimum of 130 grams of carbohydrates daily. This would be the equivalent of eating a bowl of bran flakes with milk and berries in the morning, a sandwich on whole grain bread at lunch, an apple for a snack and then vegetables and brown rice for dinner. Most people exceed this amount and consume two hundred to 330 grams per day, unless they are following a low carb diet.

PROTEIN

Protein is a necessary component for building, maintaining, and repairing many bodily systems and processes. Protein is required for:

- Production of collagen and keratin, which are the structural components of bones, teeth, hair, and the outer layer of skin. Collagen and keratin maintain the structure of blood vessels;
- Production of hormones, such as insulin and thyroid hormone;
- Production of enzymes that control chemical reactions in the body;
- Production of antibodies, white blood cells and other immune factors;
- Transportation of oxygen, vitamins and minerals to target cells throughout the body; and
- Provision of a secondary source of energy when there is not enough carbohydrates available, such as when you skip a meal or follow a low carb diet.

PROTEIN FOOD SOURCES

When we eat protein it raises our metabolic rate to a greater extent than eating just carbohydrates or fat alone. And when protein is eaten with carbs it slows the blood glucose response because it slows the digestion of carbs, as does fat (although fat doesn't raise your metoblic rate).

PROTEIN TO LOWER THE GI?

Eating protein with carbohydrates in a meal can help keep insulin levels under control. This is because eating protein triggers the release of the hormone glucagon, which has the opposite effect of insulin. Glucagon helps normalize blood sugar by raising or lowering it as needed by the body.

Protein is found in animal products, nuts, legumes and to a lesser extent in fruits and vegetables. When we eat protein our body breaks it down into amino acids—some are called *essential* because they must be provided by the food we eat. Others that can be produced by the body are called *non-essential*.

Protein from animal sources contains all of the essential amino acids. Therefore your best sources of lean protein are chicken, turkey, fish and eggs. Choose free-range and organic where possible to reduce ingesting harmful hormones and chemicals.

Plant proteins do not contain all the essential amino acids and are considered *incomplete* proteins. It is possible however to combine various plant proteins to get all the essential amino acids. For example, eating oats, lentils and sunflower seeds either together or separately throughout the day provides all the essential amino acids. You could also combine whole wheat pasta with white kidney beans or tofu with brown rice to get all the necessary amino acids. It just requires careful meal planning.

There are certain advantages to eating plant over animal protein—plant proteins provide fibre and phytochemicals (antioxidants), do not contain saturated fat, and may play a role in disease prevention. Soy protein, for example, has been shown to significantly lower cholesterol and triglyceride levels, and to protect against bone loss. A number of studies have found lower risk of chronic disease in those who eat a plant-based diet.

EATING THE RIGHT AMOUNT OF PROTEIN

Studies show a low protein diet increases your risk of osteoporosis and bone fracture. A low protein diet will also decrease your body's ability to heal itself, lower immune function, slow your metabolism, and affect your memory. Too much protein in the diet increases your risk of high blood pressure, heart disease and certain cancers. The NIH recommends that protein make up fifteen to thirty-five percent of your total caloric intake.

FATS

Fat has become a negative word as it is associated with obesity, yet we do need a certain amount of fat in our diets and on our body. There are *good* fats and *bad* fats. Choosing good fats and avoiding bad fats will greatly improve your overall health and weight loss efforts.

GOOD FATS

The good fats are the unsaturated fats, namely the monounsaturated fats (olive, canola and peanut oil) and polyunsaturated fats. The polyunsaturated fats provide us with essential fatty acids (EFAs) and they are broken down into two groups. Omega-6 fatty acids: linoleic acid (LA), which is converted into gamma-linolenic acid (GLA) and arachidonic acid (AA). Omega-3 fatty acids: alpha-linolenic acid (ALA), which is converted into eicosapentaenoic acid (EPA) and docosahexaenoic acid (DHA).

The body cannot make EFAs, so they must be obtained through diet or supplementation. They are essential for many body processes and functions:

- Growing and developing brain, nervous system, adrenal glands, sex organs inner ear and eyes;
- Providing energy (fat is the most concentrated source of energy);
- Absorbing fat-soluble vitamins (vitamins A, D, E, K, and carotenoids);
- Maintaining cell membrane integrity;
- Regulating cell processes such as gene activation and expression, enzyme function and fat oxidation; and
- Producing hormones and chemical messengers.

FAT FOOD SOURCES

Here is a breakdown of the EFAs and their sources:

- LA—found in vegetable oils such as safflower, evening primrose, sunflower, corn, hemp, canola and olive oil;
- GLA—found in borage, black currant and evening primrose oils;
- AA—found in meat and eggs. We get adequate AA through diet. Too much of this fat is not good as it causes inflammation;
- ALA—found in flaxseed and hemp oil and to a smaller extent in nuts, green leafy vegetables, wheat germ and black currant seeds; and
- EPA and DHA—found in fatty fish, such as salmon, mackerel, herring, cod, sardines and tuna.

There is great controversy over what is the optimal dietary intake ratio of omega-6 to omega-3 fatty acids. It is estimated that we currently get around a fifteen to one ratio, whereas leading EFA authorities recommend a ratio closer to four to one, or even two to one.

The Institute of Medicine has set an adequate intake level for linoleic acid for adults age nineteen to fifty years at seventeen grams daily for men and twelve grams daily for women; alpha-linolenic acid at 1.6 grams daily for men and 1.1 grams daily for women. These levels are lower for younger and older individuals.

Rather than trying to calculate the perfect ratio or intake, aim to have more omega-3s (fish, flaxseed, hemp and seed oils) and GLA (borage, black current or primrose oil) from diet and/or supplements as these are the fats that are commonly deficient, yet offer a number of health benefits.

Diets rich in the omega-3 fatty acids offer cardio protection by lowering blood cholesterol and triglyceride levels, reducing blood clotting, and reducing the risk of heart attack and sudden death. These fats also reduce inflammation and are helpful for arthritis and other inflammatory disorders. GLA, an omega-6 fatty acid, also reduces inflammation, and prevents clotting, dilates blood vessels, improves skin health, and benefits those with diabetes and arthritis.

BAD FATS

There are two fats that should be limited or completely avoided if possible—saturated fats and trans fats.

SATURATED FATS

Saturated fats are found in animal products such as meat, poultry, milk, cheese, butter and lard, as well as in tropical oils (such as palm, palm kernel and coconut oil) and foods made from these oils. These fats are high in cholesterol and linked to heart disease, high cholesterol, obesity and cancers of the breast, colon and prostate.

Most people get thirty-eight percent or more of the day's calories from fat while health authorities suggest no more than twenty to thirty-five percent, of which less than ten percent is saturated fat. To cut your intake of saturated fat, trim fat and skin from meat, choose lean poultry over red meat, and choose low-fat cheese and dairy (cottage cheese, feta and hard cheeses have less fat). Butter is fine in moderation.

TRANS FATS

Trans fatty acids are naturally found in small amounts in animal products. However, the majority of trans fats in our diet come from man-made foods. Trans fats are created when oils undergo a chemical process called hydrogenation, which changes them into a solid form. This is the process that turns vegetable oil into margarine. Trans fat is also found in cookies, crackers, french fries, baked goods and other snack foods.

When trans fats were first introduced into our food supply they were thought to be a healthier alternative to saturated fats. Many years later this was found to be false. Trans fats elevate cholesterol levels, increasing the risk for heart disease and heart attack, and are also linked to cancer, particularly breast cancer. The Institute of Medicine has stated that there is no safe limit for trans fats in the diet and that we should reduce consumption of these dangerous fats. Food companies have been making efforts in this area. You will now see many packaged foods labelled "trans fat free."

CHOLESTEROL

Cholesterol is a waxy substance found in the fats (lipids) in our blood. It is manufactured in the liver and also obtained from consuming saturated and trans fats.

Approximately seventy-five percent of the body's cholesterol is produced in the liver, the rest is obtained from diet. While having elevated blood cholesterol levels is a risk factor for heart disease, the news on cholesterol is not all bad—the body requires it to produce sex hormones, maintain cell membranes, and for a healthy nervous system.

In addition to diet, cholesterol levels can also be elevated by family history (genetics), lack of activity, stress and liver disorders.

As with fats, there is good and bad when it comes to cholesterol. The good cholesterol is HDL (high density lipoproteins) and the bad is LDL (low density lipoproteins). LDL cholesterol can build up in the artery walls of the brain and heart, narrowing the passageways for blood flow—a process known as atherosclerosis, the precursor to heart disease and stroke.

HDL cholesterol is called good cholesterol because it picks up the LDL deposited in the arteries and transports it to the liver to be broken down and eliminated.

To help lower LDL and raise HDL levels, exercise regularly, minimize saturated fats, avoid trans fats, and don't smoke (smoking lowers HDL).

TRIGLYCERIDES

Triglycerides (TG) are the form in which most fats exist. They are also present in the blood along with cholesterol.

A diet that is high in fat, sugar, refined carbohydrates and alcohol can elevate TGs. Overeating also raises TG levels because excess calories are converted to fat in the liver and then into TGs to be transported in the blood. High levels of triglycerides are associated with heart disease and diabetes. It is possible for triglycerides to be high even when blood cholesterol is normal, so get your levels checked regularly. In most cases, TG levels can be effectively managed with diet and exercise.

THE GI IS ONLY THE BEGINNING

Now that we have an understanding of the glycemic index, the role of insulin, and our nutritional needs, it's time to look at how and why the glycemic index can be an effective tool for achieving optimal health and weight loss.

First and foremost, I want to reiterate that eating according to glycemic index alone does not ensure optimal health or successful weight loss. The glycemic index works for weight loss and overall health only when used as one aspect of an overall health strategy. In order to lose weight and decrease your risk of chronic disease, you need to eat a diet that is low in saturated fats and trans fats and includes plenty of lean protein, healthy carbohydrates such as whole-grains, legumes, fruits and vegetables and a balanced supply of healthy fats. Watching your portion size and getting regular exercise are also critical for long-term health and weight management.

Since a variety of factors affect the glycemic load of a meal, the glycemic value of individual foods is not the only consideration. Nevertheless, what the glycemic index does offer is help in choosing what type of carbohydrate to eat. The bottom line is healthy eating and using the GI as a guide helps narrow down the carbohydrate choices. Among the multiple carbohydrate options available, the glycemic index, when followed with common sense, helps us choose foods with the "right" carbohydrates and this in turn, due to its numerous positive effects on blood sugar, increases our chances of achieving optimal health.

5
CHAPTER
Nutritional Strategies

In order to achieve weight-loss success and improved blood sugar control, you need to develop a comprehensive strategy that includes a balanced diet, consistent exercise and safe supplementation. When you're ready to do it, you need to make a commitment to lifelong changes. Changing your diet and lifestyle for a month or two is a great start, but it is not enough to reduce your risk of disease and increase your lifelong vitality. For long-term success, you need to make long-term changes. I believe that part of those changes must include an awareness of the glycemic index and the impact of blood sugar on health. By making the effort to adopt a healthier diet, including low GI foods, and by adopting a more active lifestyle, you can achieve phenomenal health rewards. These include weight loss, improved energy and physical fitness, better blood sugar control and lower blood pressure and cholesterol levels, and a reduced risk of chronic disease.

A healthy, balanced diet is key for effective weight management. But what exactly does that mean? Recall from the previous section that the Institute of Medicine recommends that adults receive the following:

- Forty-five to sixty-five percent of their calories from carbohydrates
- twenty to thirty-five percent from fat
- fifteen to thirty-five percent from protein

Since carbohydrates, fat and protein all serve as energy sources and provide calories, these ranges should be used as a guideline for menu planning. The question is which foods should comprise these calories? Unless you're choosing healthy foods low on the glycemic index for the vast majority of your meals, your efforts to lose weight and keep it off will not yield the results you want. There is no short cut or "magic bullet." Experts agree that healthy eating on a daily basis rather than short-term restrictive dieting is the best way to lose weight and keep it off. Considerable research indicates that following the glycemic index can also help blood sugar balancing and improve overall well-being. So, with this in mind, here are ten tips for winning at weight loss with the glycemic index:

1. Learn Your Glycemic Index by Heart

Okay...that might sound like a lot of work, but it's really not. Start by looking through the GI value chart following this section. Look for foods you like to eat and see whether they are low, moderate or high GI. Try to remember the GI value of foods when meal planning. As often as possible, choose low GI foods. Moderate GI foods should be eaten in moderation and avoid high GI whenever possible. Keep a copy of the food value chart handy, on your fridge and in your purse, to refer to when grocery shopping, cooking, or dining out.

2. Reach for Fruits and Vegetables First

Fresh, natural, unprocessed fruits and vegetables should form the basis of your diet. They are naturally low GI, especially dark green vegetables, apples, pears and berries. This tip may seem obvious but it's the hardest one to implement, especially when you are tired, cold, hungry or feeling blue. Furthermore, the typical Western diet includes so many high GI foods (often called "comfort foods"), that it will take a while to train yourself to reach for fruits and veggies first.

3. Choose Quality, Low GI Carbohydrates

Remember that this is not a low carb diet. The glycemic index allows you to choose a wide variety of carbohydrates at every meal. By choosing low GI carbs, you will attain a more balanced diet, increase feelings of satiety after a meal and achieve better blood sugar control.

Choose whole-grains over refined and processed products. Refined grains, such as white bread, white pasta, crackers, processed cereals, rice cakes, pretzels and bagels, have most of the vitamins, minerals and fiber found in the outer layer stripped away during the refinement process. These foods are nothing more than "empty calories" as they are often high in sugar and calories but low in nutritional value. If you enjoy these foods, reserve them as a special treat and minimize the serving size. Also, make sure to limit your intake of starchy carbs such as potatoes.

Instead, look at keeping your pantry stocked with low GI carbs including different types of beans (chick peas, lentils), sweet potatoes, sourdough, pita or whole grain sprouted breads and whole grain English muffins, oatmeal, muesli or rolled oat cereals, whole wheat or spinach pasta, basmati or whole grain brown rice, and plenty of fruits and vegetables (including carrots, which have been given a bad reputation due to some misleading research).

4. Always Include Protein and Healthy Fats in Every Meal

Proteins and fats are essential to a healthy, balanced diet, and also help to lower the glycemic impact of any given meal.

Protein is vital for building and maintaining lean muscle mass. Without adequate protein, dieting and exercise can cause the body to burn muscle for fuel

FILL UP ON FIBER

Most North Americans only consume about ten to fifteen grams of fiber daily, a fraction of the recommended twenty-five to thirty-eight grams daily for adults. Dietary fiber is a powerful asset to anyone trying to lose body fat. Fiber increases satiety; it makes us feel more full because it slows digestion. Dietary fiber also helps balance blood sugar and insulin levels, and improves digestion and elimination.

Dietary fiber is found in fruits, vegetables, beans, seeds and whole-grains, such as wheat and oat bran. If your diet is lacking in fiber, look for a supplement. When increasing your fiber intake, do it gradually to minimize temporary gas or bloating that occurs in the early stages of increasing fiber intake.

and this can result in a lowering of your basal metabolic rate—the rate at which you burn calories. Focus on eating lean protein, such as poultry, fish, eggs, nuts, seeds and tofu. Red meat is okay in moderation, but make sure to trim the fat. If following a vegetarian diet, be sure to incorporate a variety of plant-based proteins to ensure all essential amino acids are consumed. If you can't get enough protein in your diet, consider a protein supplement that provides at least twenty grams per serving, is low in carbohydrate and free of artificial ingredients and sweeteners.

As discussed in Chapter 4, a certain amount of good fats (essential fatty acids) are required for health. Choose quality sources of fats including fish, nuts and seeds, and milled flax and hemp seed. Avoid saturated and trans fats, which are found in processed and fast foods. These fats are high in calories—providing nine calories per gram compared to only four calories per gram with protein and carbohydrates—low in nutritional value, and research has linked diets high in these fats to heart disease and cancer. Plus these fats fill you up more slowly because they take longer to metabolize and digest. Avoid the fat-free frenzy because many of the fat-free products (such as sour cream and yogurt) use sugar or starch in place of fat and end up providing just as many or more calories as the original product.

BUTTER VS. MARGARINE

Butter contains saturated fats, however they are short-chain saturates, which are easily digested and provide a source of usable energy. Butter also contains nutrients: lecithin, vitamins A and E and selenium. Most margarines contain hydrogenated oils (trans fats), which are man-made processed fats that are linked to heart disease and cancer. The exception is non-hydrogenated margarines, such as Becel™, which contain beneficial plant sterols that can help lower cholesterol. So the bottom line is, choose butter or a non-hydrogenated margarine.

5. Enjoy a Variety of Wholesome Foods

To get a broad range of nutrients in your diet, enjoy a variety of foods, rather than sticking to your favourites. We have a tendency to eat the same foods over and over. By doing this we miss out on some of the nutrients provided by eating different foods. This is particularly important with vegetables and fruits as their nutrient profiles vary greatly, even among low to moderate GI fruits and vegetables. To obtain the many antioxidants, vitamins, minerals, and phytonutrients eat a variety of plant foods every day. Experiment with new foods and recipes, and try to reintroduce previously disliked foods.

READING FOOD LABELS AND CALCULATING CALORIES

Macronutrients provide us with calories as follows:

Carbohydrate—four calories per gram

Protein—four calories per gram

Fat—nine calories per gram

If a food product contains ten grams carbohydrate, two grams protein and one gram fat per serving, it would provide $10 \times 4 = 40$ calories from carbohydrate, $2 \times 4 = 8$ calories from protein, and $1 \times 9 = 9$ calories from fat for a total calorie count of 57 calories per serving.

---

6. Avoid Portion Distortion

Overeating can lead to obesity, high triglycerides, insulin resistance, free radical damage and shortened life expectancy. To prevent overeating, control your portion sizes and eat slowly. A serving equals one piece of fruit, one cup of raw or ½ cup cooked vegetables, one slice of bread, ½ cup of cooked rice or pasta, or two to three ounces of meat. Eating slowly allows your stomach to send a message to your brain that you are full. Chew your food thoroughly and drink water to allow for proper digestion. It should take you twenty to thirty minutes to eat a meal.

Caloric requirements are dependent upon your age, gender, height, weight and activity level. Here are averages for ages thirty years and older.

Height/Weight	Gender	Calories (Sedentary)	Calories (Active)
5'1" 98 to 132 pounds	Women	1688 – 1834	2104 – 2290
	Men	1919 – 2167	2104 – 2290
5'5" 111 to 150 pounds	Women	1816 – 1982	2267 – 2477
	Men	2068 – 2349	2490 – 2842
5'9" 125 to 169 pounds	Women	1948 – 2134	2434 – 2670
	Men	2222 – 2538	2683 – 3078
6'1" 139 to 188 pounds	Women	2083 – 2290	2605 – 2869
	Men	2382 – 2736	2883 – 3325

- Source: The Institute of Medicine (IOM)
- Please consult your primary healthcare provider if pregnant, lactating or engaged in vigorous physical activity.

7. EAT SMALL FREQUENT MEALS

Try to eat every three hours: three small meals and two snacks daily. This will improve metabolism (calorie burning) and blood sugar balance, which improves energy and mood.

Breakfast is essential to fuel your body. If you aren't very hungry in the morning, then have a light meal such as yogurt and berries or a protein shake. Try not to eat too late in the evening (after 8pm) as this could impact sleep. Don't skip meals, even if trying to lose weight, since this causes fatigue, poor concentration, sluggish metabolism and triggers food cravings. When you are hungry between meals, snack on healthy, low GI foods, such as fruit, yogurt, raw vegetables, nuts and seeds.

8. GO EASY ON SALT

Salt (sodium) is necessary for health as it helps maintain fluid balance and aids muscle and nerve function. However, most of the sodium in the typical Western diet comes from the salt shaker and from processed and prepared foods, such as deli meats, condiments (ketchup), dressings and sauces (soy) and snack foods (chips, pretzels). A high sodium diet is unhealthy and causes fluid retention, meaning it can contribute to water weight gain. Many people consume far more salt than required, and this can contribute to high blood pressure, especially in older individuals, African Americans and those with diabetes and kidney disease. So cut back on these foods and season with herbs or flavoured oils and vinegars rather than the salt shaker.

TIP: To add more zing to your meals, add fresh lemon juice or apple cider vinegar, which can lower the glycemic value of a meal by up to thirty percent.

9. WATCH YOUR CAFFEINE AND ALCOHOL INTAKE

If you drink caffeinated beverages or alcohol, do so in moderation. Limit your intake to no more than two cups of caffeine daily. A high intake of caffeine can promote calcium loss from bones, increase blood pressure, affect fertility in women and cause sleep disturbances (insomnia), irritability, anxiety, and tremors. Black tea and green tea contain some caffeine but it is blunted by an amino acid (theanine), which has a calming effect. Be on the lookout for hidden caffeine. Cola contains about thirty-five milligrams of caffeine per can. Chocolate contains six to twenty milligrams per thirty gram piece (one ounce).

Heavy and chronic drinking is linked to a number of health concerns, including liver and cardiovascular disease, and malnutrition. Plus, alcohol floods the body with empty calories. Depending on the beverage, it provides anywhere from twenty to 124 calories per ounce. Moderate alcohol consumption, no more than two glasses per day of red wine and dark beers, however, can reduce the risk of heart disease, likely due to its antioxidant content.

10. Set Manageable Goals for Yourself

Give yourself time to incorporate your new way of eating into your lifestyle. Remember, it took a lifetime to develop these eating habits and it won't take a few short months to rid you of them completely. This will be a work in progress that may take as long as a year to fall into a comfortable rhythm. To start, look at a three-month timeline:

- Month one is your adjustment period. Be kind to yourself and experiment as much as possible as you adjust from your old way of eating to your new way.
- Month two should see this new way of eating become a habit. During this month, be disciplined about sticking to your new eating habits. Discover where you have challenges, such as being too busy on weeknights to cook, and develop strategies to deal with these challenges.
- During month three you should start to see noticeable improvements to your health, blood sugar and weight. If you are not seeing appreciable changes, seek expert advice.

If you're not making headway by the end of month three, consider hiring a professional for some expert tips to get you moving in the right direction.

- Registered Dietitian—book an appointment with a registered dietitian to help identify your problem areas and learn strategies to overcome them. It may take no more than one appointment to get things straightened out. Keep a food journal before your first appointment.
- Naturopath (or complementary health care provider)—a wholistic health care provider can work with you to identify problems such as nutritional deficiencies or food allergies that may be impacting your ability to lose weight and stick to a new eating style.
- Counsellor—if your relationship with food seems like it's not in your control, you may be suffering from compulsive or emotional eating. Expert advice could help you overcome this obstacle.

Glycemic Index Food Value Chart

Try to choose low and moderate GI foods more often and eat high GI foods only occasionally and in smaller portions.

Here are some tips to help you lower the glycemic impact of your daily meals:

- While certain foods might register as low GI (for example, Italian ice cream or certain chocolate bars), they should only be eaten in moderation or as an occasional treat because these foods are high in saturated fat and calories.
- Try to choose at least one low GI food at each meal. If you choose a high GI food, combine it with a low GI food, for an overall medium GI meal.

LOW GLYCEMIC (55 or less)

Apples/apple juice
Apricots (dried)
Banana (ripe)
Barley
Beans (haricot, lima, kidney,
  mung, navy and pinto)
Bean sprouts
Broccoli
Carrots (raw)
Cereals (All-Bran™)
Chapati (bread)
Cherries
Chickpeas
Chocolate (dark)
Grapefruit
Grapes
Kiwi fruit
Lentils
Milk
Oat bran bread
Oatmeal (slow-cook oats)
Oranges
Pasta al dente (firm)
Peaches
Pears
Peppers
Plums
Pumpernickel bread
Rice (long grain, brown,
  converted, wild)
Sourdough bread
Soybeans
Soy beverages
Split peas
Sushi
Sweet potatoes
Syrup (pure maple)
Taro
Yam
Yogurt (plain)

MODERATE GLYCEMIC (56 to 69)

Arrowroot biscuit
Beer
Beets (canned)
Breton crackers
Brown rice
Buckwheat
Cantaloupe
Cereal (Shredded
  Wheat™, Just Right™,
  Nutrigrain and Raisin
  Bran™)
Corn (sweet)
Cornmeal
Couscous
Cranberry Juice Coctail
Croissant (white)
Dried fruit (mixed)
Hamburger bun (white)
Honey
Jam (strawberry)
Mango (ripe)
Muesli
New potatoes
Pancakes
Papaya
Pasta (white)
Pineapple
Pita bread
Popcorn
Porridge (rolled oats)
Raisins
Rice (basmati)
Rye bread
Split pea/green pea soup
Sugar (sucrose)
Taco shells (corn)
Wheat Thins™
Whole wheat bread

HIGH GLYCEMIC (70 and over)

Bagel (white)
Baked white potato
Bread stuffing
Broad beans
Candy (sugar)
Cereal (Cheerios™,
  Crispix™, CornFlakes™,
  Corn Pops™,
  Grapenuts™, Rice
  Krispies™, Total™)
Corn cakes (puffed)
Corn chips
Digestive cookies
Donuts
Dried dates
French baguette
French fries
Fruit Roll-Ups®
Glucose
Graham wafers
Instant mashed potatoes
Jellybeans
Kaiser roll
Life Savers®
Parsnips
Pasta (corn, rice)
Pop-Tarts™
Pretzels
Rice (instant, jasmine)
Rice bread
Rice cakes (white)
Rice crackers
Rutabagas
Snack chips
Soda crackers
Sports drinks
Tapioca (boiled)
Watermelon
White bread

- Base your food choices primarily on overall nutrition and include vitamins, minerals and fiber. Don't dismiss healthy foods such as dried dates, watermelon or mangos because they have a high GI. Other nutritional benefits make them good choices. Plus, remember that fruits and vegetables tend to have a low to moderate glycemic load because the amount of carbohydrates per serving is a factor. For example, a mango has a GI of sixty (moderate) but provides fifteen grams of carbohydrate per serving. Therefore the glycemic load is (60 X 15) ÷ 100 = 9.1 (a low value). Just eat in moderation and watch your portion sizes— eating one mango won't have a dramatic effect on your blood sugar, but eating two or three most definitely will. Likewise, don't indulge in excessive amounts of low GI foods simply because they are low GI. Calories still count.
- Incorporate more spices to add flavour to your meals. Use cinnamon as a low GI way to sweeten a variety of foods such as yogurt, coffee and whole grain toast.
- If you are diabetic, monitor your blood glucose level before eating and one to two hours afterwards to see different meal combinations impact your body. Keep a mental or written journal of what works for you and what doesn't.

FUNCTIONAL FOODS

Functional foods, as defined by the International Food Information Council, are "foods that offer health benefits beyond basic nutrition." In other words, these foods provide more than just vitamins and minerals—they contain compounds that have beneficial actions in the body and can reduce the risk of chronic disease. These are foods that you want to include more of in your daily diet. Here are my top five recommended functional foods. Try to include at least one of these functional foods in your diet each day.

1. BERRIES

Berries, cherries and red grapes contain plant pigments called anthocyanidins, which have antioxidant properties, preventing free radical damage and reducing the risk of chronic disease. These compounds are also important for proper brain and blood vessel function. Cranberries contain proanthocyanidins, which have been shown to reduce the risk of urinary tract infections. Preliminary research also shows that these compounds may help lower cholesterol, improve gum health, prevent ulcers and prevent brain damage after a stroke. Berries and grapes have a low GI.

2. DEEP GREEN VEGETABLES

Collard greens and kale contain plant pigments called lutein and zeaxanthin, which are important for eye health and can reduce the risk of macular degeneration (age-related blindness). One to two servings of kale or collard greens per week provide the recommended amount of lutein and zeaxanthin. Broccoli contains sulphoraphane and indole-3 carbinol, two antioxidants that neutralize free radicals, enhance detoxification and may reduce the risk of cancer.

3. Fish

Fish oils contain omega-3 fatty acids (EPA and DHA) which have been found to reduce risk of CHD. Specifically they reduce triglycerides, increase HDL (good cholesterol), reduce inflammation, prevent clotting and reduce blood pressure. They are also known to be beneficial for visual function and brain health.

4. Garlic

Garlic contains sulphur compounds that offer a number of health benefits. Studies have shown that garlic mildly reduces cholesterol, reduces LDL oxidation (atherosclerosis), prevents blood clotting, reduces the risk of diabetes, and fights infections and cancer. Studies have found benefits with as little as nine hundred milligrams of garlic per day, which is approximately equivalent to one clove.

5. Yogurt

Yogurt contains active bacteria cultures, known as probiotics or friendly bacteria, which improve gastrointestinal health (digestion and elimination) and immune function. These active cultures also help digest the naturally occurring sugar (lactose) in dairy products that causes bloating and diarrhea in some people. Look for plain, unsweetened yogurt, and avoid the "diet" or "light" yogurts, since they are sweetened with aspartame.

Why Water Works

One of the most important dietary tips I can give you is actually a simple one—drink plenty of pure water daily. Drinking water is critical for weight loss and for supporting overall health. While you are losing weight, toxins stored in the fat tissue are released into your bloodstream. Drinking plenty of pure water makes it easier for your liver and kidneys to eliminate toxins. Water also works with fiber to keep your bowels regular and prevent constipation. Feeling thirsty is a sign of dehydration, and this sign is sometimes confused with hunger. Drinking water throughout the day will keep you hydrated, and prevent dehydration. Having a glass before and during meals can also help fill you up and reduce the quantity of food consumed.

The National Research Council recommends that adults consume four cups or one liter of water for every one thousand calories utilized by physical activity. If the average woman burns 2,200 calories per day, then she would need to drink nine cups of water per day. You should consume more water if you are pregnant, breastfeeding or engaging in vigorous physical exercise. Children should also try to drink at least eight glasses of water each day.

6
CHAPTER

Let's Get Physical

Regular exercise is an important aspect of glycemic control, says a report from the Ottawa Health Research Institute in Canada. These researchers did a comprehensive review of clinical studies that looked at the effects of at least eight weeks of exercise on adults with Type 2 diabetes. They found fourteen trials that met their criteria, and from those studies, determined that regular exercise did in fact reduce the risk of diabetic complications by lowering blood sugar levels.

Our modern way of life with automated, drive-through, express convenience, however, offers few opportunities for regular exercise. While you can certainly lose weight by reducing your calorie intake, regular exercise can greatly enhance your weight-loss program. Consider this: adding a thirty-minute brisk walk four days a week, can double your rate of weight loss. Boost that to five days a week and the rewards are greater. Those who work out five times a week have been found to lose three times as much fat as those who exercise only two or three times weekly.

There are many reasons why exercise is so helpful for weight loss. First, it boosts metabolism (the rate of calorie burning). In fact, your basal (resting) metabolic rate is heightened for four to twenty-four hours after vigorous physical activity. Secondly, exercise builds strong, healthy muscles and muscle burns more calories than any other part of the body. One pound of muscle burns approximately fifty calories per day, compared to a pound of fat, which burns only two to three calories per day. Thirdly, exercise slows down the passage of food through the digestive tract, so that your stomach takes longer to empty and you feel full longer. Exercise also helps balance blood sugar levels by pulling stored calories (energy) from glucose and fat out of tissues. In this way, blood glucose levels stay balanced and you are less likely to feel hungry.

The benefits of exercise extend to so many other aspects of health. Consider these other impressive benefits:

- Increased strength—the National Institutes of Health found that men and women, between the ages of eighty-six and ninety-six, tripled the muscular strength of their legs when they worked out with weights.

- Improved energy—believe it or not, regular exercise can actually make you feel more energized.
- Improved mood—even light exercise can boost your emotional well-being. Aerobic exercise stimulates the release of certain mood-elevating compounds called endorphins, "feel good" chemicals. These natural painkillers induce relaxation and relieve depression.
- Increased mental acuity—physical activity can invigorate and revitalize the mind and improve the flow of blood, oxygen and nutrients to all the body's organs, including the brain.
- Better sleep—studies have shown that exercise can improve sleep quality.
- Pain relief—exercise triggers the release of pain-reducing endorphins. Strength training and stretching can help decrease arthritis pain and improve joint flexibility.
- Increased bone density—activities that put stress on the bones (walking, weight training) stimulate bone growth and protect against bone loss. In one study, sedentary ninety-year-old nursing home residents performed mild exercises for thirty minutes, three times a week. On average, they experienced a 4.2 percent increase in their bone density.
- Reduced risk of diabetes—exercise improves blood sugar balance and insulin resistance, and has been shown in many studies to reduce the risk of Type 2 diabetes. It can also benefit those with diabetes, and may reduce the need for medication and/or insulin.
- Reduced risk of heart disease—in a study conducted at Washington University School of Medicine in St. Louis, a group of individuals participated in a twelve-month exercise program that increased their cardiovascular function by twenty-five to thirty percent. Exercise can also effectively lower blood pressure and cholesterol, and facilitate weight loss, reducing risk factors for heart disease.
- Enhanced longevity—regular physical activity lowers the risk of death from all causes.

CREATING YOUR EXERCISE PROGRAM

If you have been sedentary all your life, the prospect of getting active may be intimidating. The most important advice for beginners is to take it slowly. Where do you start? Three words: just start moving. That may sound like an oversimplification but it's amazing how hard it is to make it happen. You need to look at exercise like you do other essential daily routines such as brushing your teeth, showering or cleaning up after dinner. Getting into shape is a gradual, incremental process. If you do too much too soon, you may injure yourself or become too discouraged to continue. For example, start by taking a five-minute walk. The next day, walk six or seven minutes. Day by day, steadily increase the time and intensity of your activity. You will build your capacity for physical activity, making it easier to push yourself to the next level.

For optimal results in your weight loss program, work on accumulating one hour of moderate intensity activity each day. Aim to do a combination of cardiovascular, aerobic and stretching activities. Here is a breakdown of each of these activities and some guidelines to consider:

CARDIOVASCULAR (AEROBIC) EXERCISE

Cardiovascular activities are those which involve large muscle groups and increase heart rate for more than a few minutes. Examples include brisk walking, swimming, biking, aerobics, dancing and rollerblading. These exercises help burn calories, and also improve cardiovascular and respiratory (lung) function by conditioning the lungs to be able to use more oxygen while increasing your heart's efficiency.

Aim for thirty minutes to an hour five times per week. Pick activities you enjoy and do them in the morning or right after work, preferably on an empty stomach. Morning is best because you will have more energy and will continue to burn calories for several hours afterward.

To increase intensity, add resistance or power to the movements. For example, when a brisk walk becomes easy, add hand weights or walk up hills. Moving your arms above your heart will also increase your heart rate.

CHECK YOUR HEART RATE

Aerobic activity should increase your heart rate to sixty to eighty percent of your maximum rate for 30 minutes or longer. To find your maximum rate, subtract your age from 220.

> For example if you are fifty years old:
> 220 – 50 = 170
> sixty to eighty percent of 170 = 102 to 136

Divide by six to get the ten-second heart beat count.

Sixty to eighty percent of 170 is seventeen to twenty-three beats every ten seconds. For optimum aerobic benefits keep your heart rate between 102 to 136 beats per minute for thirty minutes.

RESISTANCE TRAINING

Activities that challenge your muscles against resistance increase strength, endurance, and muscle mass and strengthen bones. This can be achieved with weight-lifting, exercise machines, bands/tubes, using your own body weight or lifting heavy objects. These activities are particularly important for older adults because they help prevent and slow the muscle and bone loss that occurs with aging.

Try to spend twenty to thirty minutes three to four times a week doing resistance activities. Choose two body parts per workout. For example, do chest and triceps on Monday, back and biceps on Wednesday, and legs and shoulders on Friday. Pick two exercises per body part and do two or three sets of eight to twelve repetitions of that exercise. Vary your activities and routine to continually challenge your muscles.

STRETCHING

Stretching after a workout is a great way to improve flexibility and joint health and prevent next-day soreness. Spend about five to ten minutes stretching all your muscles. Stretch slowly and gently, breathe deeply, and hold each position for at least ten seconds.

HOW MUCH EXERCISE DO I NEED?

Guidelines from the National Academy of Sciences and the Institute of Medicine (used in Canada and the United States) recommend that, regardless of weight, adults and children should spend a total of at least one hour each day in moderately intense physical activity. This recommendation takes into consideration the increased caloric intake of our population, our lack of activity, and our rising prevalence of obesity.

BUILDING ACTIVITY INTO YOUR DAY

If you don't have an hour that you can dedicate to exercise, work on incorporating more activity into your daily routine. Every little bit helps. Studies have actually shown that the benefits of exercise are cumulative (i.e. performing a few minutes of exercise at a time is equally effective as performing all the exercise at once). Here are some suggestions:

- Do housework or gardening with vim and vigour
- Take the stairs instead of the elevator
- Use your break at work to go for a brisk walk
- Ride your bike to the store
- Park your car further away and walk to your destination
- Wash your car (instead of using the drive-through)

TAKE PRIDE IN YOUR PROGRESS

Even modest weight loss can yield impressive health benefits. A weight loss of even five to ten percent has been shown to help prevent diabetes, reduce blood pressure and cholesterol, and improve quality of life.

Before you start an exercise program talk with your doctor, especially if you have any health conditions or are taking medication. If you are unfamiliar with exercise equipment or need help designing a routine tailored to your needs, consult with a certified personal trainer. Don't expect overnight results. Set reasonable goals, be consistent with your exercises and your will see both the physical and emotional rewards. Since motivation is critical, consider getting a workout partner, vary your activities, and most importantly—have fun.

7
CHAPTER

Sleep and De-Stress for Success

Adequate sleep and stress management are essential, but often overlooked factors that are paramount for physical and emotional well-being and successful weight loss. Let's take a closer look at how these factors impact our ability to lose weight.

SLEEP

Sleep is one of our body's most basic needs, yet with today's busy lifestyles sleep deprivation has become all too common. In fact, nearly half of all adults report having difficulty sleeping. While we think of sleep as a relaxing and passive state, there is actually quite a lot going on in our bodies during sleep. The exact amount of sleep needed varies among individuals, but is thought to be between seven and nine hours. Getting less than six hours is associated with health problems such as memory loss, poor concentration, depression, headache, irritability, increased response to stress, high blood pressure, depressed immune function and low libido.

Recently, sleep deprivation has been linked to obesity. Several studies have shown that getting less than six hours per night can lead to hormonal changes that reduce metabolism and increase appetite—factors that lead to weight gain. Specifically, lack of sleep increases the level of a hormone called ghrelin, which increases appetite. Lack of sleep also reduces levels of another hormone, called human growth hormone, and this leads to a reduced metabolism. In one study, participants who slept five hours per night were seventy-three percent more likely to become obese than those getting seven to nine nightly hours of sleep. So for better appetite and weight control, don't skimp on sleep.

To improve your sleep, develop a good bedtime routine. Going to bed at approximately the same time each night is recommended. Make your bedroom quiet, comfortable and dark and used for sleep only (don't work in bed). Do relaxing activities in the evening—read a book, have a warm bath or meditate.

DID YOU KNOW...

Eating before bedtime may result in poor sleep habits. Snacking before bedtime, especially on refined carbohydrates, will raise insulin levels. Raised insulin levels can prevent the action of melatonin, the sleep-inducing hormone. Lack of sleep, particularly deep (delta) sleep not only makes us feel tired, but also has serious consequences—memory loss, poor concentration, depression, headache, irritability, increased response to stress, high blood pressure, depressed immune function and low libido. More recently sleep deprivation has been linked to obesity due to hormonal changes that reduce metabolism and increase appetite.

STRESS

Stress is a primary cause of many health problems today. According to recent reports forty-three percent of all adults suffer the adverse health effects of stress, and stress-related ailments account for seventy-five to ninety percent of all visits to physicians. Stress is not an external force but rather how we react to external pressures. During stress, the body releases stress hormones—adrenaline, noradrenaline and cortisol—to prepare the body to fight, hence this is known as the fight-flight response. Heart rate, blood pressure and lung function increase to enhance the function of the heart and lungs. Numerous studies have linked stress to heart disease, cancer, diabetes, high cholesterol and blood pressure, anxiety, depression, memory loss, insomnia, muscle tension, obesity, fatigue, low libido, erectile dysfunction and menstrual cycle disturbances.

In recent years, many studies have looked at the connection between stress and obesity. Researchers have found that chronic stress causes weight gain due to a number of factors. Chronic stress increases the production of cortisol—a hormone that promotes fat storage, primarily around the belly. Stress also triggers cravings for carbohydrates and sweets. Lastly, stress can lead to muscle wasting, which reduces metabolism.

For weight-loss success, work on reducing your stress. Start by identifying your stressors and then look at ways that you can change your reaction to those situations. It may be a matter of analyzing and rethinking your natural reaction, avoiding certain situations or utilizing one of the following stress-reducing strategies:

• Meditation—sit down in a quiet area and close your eyes. Relax all your muscles, starting with your feet and working up. Clear your mind and focus your attention on your breathing or a calming sight or sound. Breathe in slowly and deeply, and then exhale out. Do this for ten or twenty minutes once or twice daily.

• Visualization—close your eyes, take a few deep breaths, and visualize a picture or event that made you feel calm and centered. Focus on the details, sounds, images and smells.

- Body therapies—try massage, acupuncture and acupressure to promote relaxation of the body and mind.
- Supplements—choose ones that help reduce stress such as theanine, B-vitamins and magnesium.
- Boundaries—learn to say "no". Taking on too much leads to feeling overwhelmed and pressed for time.
- Avoid negativity—negative people, places and events can create stress.
- Talk about it—share your feelings and concerns and get support from friends, family or a therapist.

Lack of sleep and stress can certainly take a toll on your body and mind, so it is absolutely crucial to find ways to improve your sleep patterns and cope effectively with stress.

8

CHAPTER

Nutritional Supplements

Without a doubt, proper eating and regular exercise are the cornerstones for healthy, long-term weight loss and improved blood sugar control. However, certain nutritional supplements can offer significant benefits and provide support during challenging times. Finding the right supplement can help the following:

- Help control blood sugar
- Neutralize carbohydrates
- Prevent the storage of fat
- Enhance your metabolism
- Promote lean muscle mass
- Curb your appetite
- Control sugar cravings

While the shelves of pharmacies and health food stores are lined with weight-loss products, few are clinically tested for safety and efficacy. As a pharmacist, my number one question when a new product hits the market is, has it undergone clinical tests? I'm pleased to say that there are a handful of supplements, which in clinical studies are shown to offer various benefits.

PHASE 2®

Phase 2 is a standardized extract derived from the white kidney bean that promotes weight loss and improves glycemic control by neutralizing ingested starches. In clinical studies, Phase 2 has been shown to lower blood sugar levels after a meal, reduce the amount of starch absorbed from starchy meals and promote loss of body fat. Phase 2 works in the intestine by temporarily inhibiting the activity of alpha amylase, the enzyme that breaks down starch into smaller glucose (sugar) molecules. As a result, fewer starch calories are absorbed from a meal and it reduces the rise in blood sugar that occurs after eating starchy foods.

RESEARCH ON PHASE 2

Several studies have examined the benefits of Phase 2. In two preliminary human studies, subjects were given a standardized meal containing sixty grams of starch (four slices of white bread) and either placebo or fifteen hundred grams of Phase 2 in a margarine spread. Postprandial (after meal) blood sugar levels were measured as an index of starch absorption. Participants who were given Phase 2 had an average sixty-six percent reduction in after-meal blood sugar levels compared to the placebo group. Participants given Phase 2 reported no adverse side effects in either study.

An independent study conducted in Italy was the first to show that supplementing with Phase 2 could lead to substantial weight loss. This double-bind, placebo-controlled study involved sixty overweight individuals aged twenty-five to forty-five. Participants were instructed to consume starchy foods during one of the principle meals, and to take their test product (Phase 2 or placebo) at that time. Researchers measured body weight, body fat percentage and hip, waist and thigh circumference at baseline and at the end of the thirty-day study period. Participants who took the Phase 2 lost an average of 6.5 pounds and 10.5 percent fat mass and had significant reductions in all body measurements compared to those in the placebo group had small and non-significant changes.

A study conducted at Northridge Hospital Medical Center, UCLA, and published in *Alternative Medicine Review*, found that participants given Phase 2 lost an average of four pounds in eight weeks, and experienced an average twenty-six-point reduction in triglycerides and greater energy. In comparison, those participants given placebo lost only 1.6 pounds.

Other weight loss studies with Phase 2 have been conducted in Mexico, Japan and the United States, yielding impressive and significant results. And most recently, Phase 2 was shown to reduce the glycemic index of white bread, which is not surprising considering that it reduces the breakdown of starch into sugar. The clinical evidence on Phase 2 is so significant that the FDA allows it to be sold with a claim for weight control.

Phase 2 is particularly helpful for those struggling with both obesity and diabetes, or those looking to improve glycemic control and insulin resistance. It allows people to eat starchy foods, while minimizing the amount of sugar absorbed. Phase 2 is safe and well tolerated and is not known to interact with any drugs or supplements. The recommended dosage of Phase 2 is 1000–1500 milligrams before starchy meals. Phase 2 is available in a variety of forms including tablets, capsules and soft chews.

FOOD INNOVATIONS

Due to the rising popularity and widespread awareness of the impact of blood sugar, companies are looking at ways of lowering the glycemic effect of traditionally high GI foods such as breads, buns and pizza crusts. One manufacturer, Pharmachem Laboratories, has developed a way to incorporate their starch neutralizer ingredient (Starchlite™) into baked good. A study at UCLA found that Starchlite substantially lowered the GI of white bread. As well, taste and texture studies have been very positive. New baked products with Starchlite are currently being developed.

PGX™

PGX (PolyGlycopleX) is a blend of highly purified, naturally-occurring, soluble fibers. In clinical studies, it has been shown to regulate after-meal blood glucose levels, increase insulin sensitivity for reduced fat storage, lower blood cholesterol, reduce appetite and food cravings and improve fat burning.

When added to liquid, PGX absorbs six hundred times its weight in water. In fact, PGX is approximately seven times as viscous as psyllium. If it is taken with adequate liquid, it will expand in the stomach and intestine and keep appetite under control for several hours by providing a sense of fullness.

RESEARCH ON PGX

The Canadian Center for Functional Medicine in Coquitlam, British Columbia, conducted a weight loss evaluation study from December 2003 through February 2004. They found that participants following their prescribed weight loss program, which included PGX, lost up to two pounds per week, primarily body fat, and maintained lean muscle mass. Besides reversing insulin resistance, PGX helps normalize important appetite hormones and cholesterol levels. Research on PGX was presented at the American Diabetes Association's annual meeting in June 2004.

The recommended dosage is two to four capsules, before meals with at least eight to sixteen ounces (240 to 480 millilitres) of water.

CINNAMON

Early studies indicate that cinnamon's bioactive compounds have health benefits. The active ingredient in cinnamon is a water-soluble polyphenol compound called MHCP. In test tube experiments, MHCP mimics insulin, activates its receptor, and works synergistically with insulin in cells.

RESEARCH ON CINNAMON

Just half a teaspoon of cinnamon a day significantly reduces blood sugar levels in diabetics, reports a 2003 study from the US Department of Agriculture's Human Nutrition Center. Volunteers with Type 2 diabetes were given one, three or six grams of cinnamon powder a day, after meals. All participants achieved blood sugar levels that were on average twenty percent lower than a control group. Some even achieved normal blood sugar levels.

Cinnulin PF® is a patented, water-soluble blend containing standardized amounts of bioactive polyphenol polymers from cinnamon. In addition to supporting healthy glucose metabolism, polyphenol polymers found in Cinnulin PF have been shown to support levels of lipids such as triglycerides, total cholesterol and low-density lipoprotein (LDL) that are already within normal ranges. Studies have shown that Cinnulin supports healthy glucose management, helps optimize healthy cholesterol levels and bolsters healthy blood pressure.

Sprinkle cinnamon on favourite foods such as yogurt, cereal or toast. Or, consider taking a cinnamon supplement, such as Cinnulin PF, which are available in health food stores and pharmacies.

CONJUGATED LINOLEIC ACID (CLA)
CLA is a derivative of linoleic acid, which is a fatty acid found naturally in certain foods, such as meat and dairy products. Supplements of CLA are made from sunflower oil. Studies have shown that CLA can improve fat metabolism and maintain or improve lean muscle mass. Specifically, it works by increasing lipolysis (fat breakdown) and enhancing fatty acid oxidation (promotes burning of fat).

Research on CLA
The most widely studied CLA product on the market is Tonalin® CLA. A one-year, double-bind study compared Tonalin CLA to placebo in 157 overweight adults. Researchers measured the participants' body fat mass and lean body mass. No changes were made to exercise or diet. At the end of the study it was found that a daily intake of 3.4 grams of Tonalin CLA produced an average nine percent reduction in body fat mass, and a small increase in lean body mass.

Subsequent to this study, 134 of the participants volunteered to continue on in order to determine the long-term safety of the product and whether they could maintain their fat loss. They continued to take a dosage of 3.4 grams of Tonalin CLA per day for an additional twelve months. There were no serious adverse effects reported and it was found that the participants were able to maintain their initial fat loss.

Most recently, a study was conducted during the holidays to determine if Tonalin could prevent the typical holiday weight gain. Forty overweight adults participated in this study that lasted for six months. The subjects were given either placebo or 3.2 grams of Tonalin CLA daily. The researchers measured body composition before, during and after the study period. Those given the Tonalin CLA lost body fat during the study period, whereas those who were given placebo gained weight. This study was published in the *International Journal of Obesity*, August 2006.

Here is a summary of some of the earlier research:

- *Journal of Nutrition* (Sept 2000)—participants taking CLA experienced an aver age reduction of five percent of body fat after twelve weeks.
- *International Journal of Obesity* (August 2001)—male subjects, classified as abdominally obese, lost an average of one inch from their waistlines in a four-week period when using CLA.
- *Lipids* (August 2001)—a study of fifty-three patients reported that those taking CLA over the fourteen-week trial experienced body fat reductions of 3.8 percent.

The recommended dosage of Tonalin is 4 grams daily, which provides 3.4 grams of actual CLA. While butter, whole milk, cheese and beef contain some CLA, it would be difficult to get the recommended amount from these foods, and consuming large amounts of them is not recommended because of their saturated fat content. CLA is well tolerated. Some studies reported increased oiliness of skin and loose stool. There are no known drug interactions.

ADVANTRA Z®

Advantra Z is a patented extract of *citrus aurantium* (bitter orange) that has been studied for its weight-loss effects. Advantra Z contains five adrenergic amines (chemicals that resemble adrenaline, especially in physiological action). These amines work together to increase thermogenesis, or the rate of calorie burning.

Citrus aurantium is chemically similar to ephedra (a once popular weight-loss aid that has been removed from the market due to serious adverse effects), but has different effects in the body. *Citrus aurantium* works by selectively stimulating beta-3 cell receptors, which are located primarily in the fatty tissue and the liver. Stimulation of these receptors activates lipolysis (fat breakdown) and thermogenesis, helping the body burn fat more efficiently. It may also give your workouts more clout. By releasing free fatty acids during aerobic exercise, this supplement may help provide more energy, thereby facilitating improved physical performance.

Research on Advantra Z

Research conducted at McGill University's Nutrition and Food Science Centre in Montreal found that Advantra Z increased the thermogenic effect of food (TEF), meaning that the subjects burned more calories and stored less fat. Researchers found a measurable increase in metabolic rate when citrus aurantium was ingested. They stated, "Furthermore, as no irregular changes in pulse pressure or blood pressure were reported, our results indicate that the alkaloid mixture is well-tolerated." Earlier studies also found that citrus aurantium had comparable thermogenic effects to ephedra, but without the side effects commonly associated with ephedra use.

There have been some concerns raised about citrus aurantium, as a few reports suggested that it could increase blood pressure. The component in citrus aurantium responsible for this effect is called synephrine. There are several forms of synephrine; Advantra-Z contains the "p" isomer, which has not been found to have any effect on blood pressure.

As well, it is important to note, that a recent evaluation of these reports revealed that most of the cases involved either ephedra alone or in combination with citrus aurantium; no direct causal relationship could be determined. Unfortunately though, media reports and misinformation fuelled unnecessary panic about Advantra Z.

In a recent study the cardiovascular effects of Advantra Z were tested on a group of twenty-three overweight adults. Subjects were given a dose of fifty-two milligrams of Advantra-Z along with 704 milligrams of caffeine and their heart rate and blood pressure were measured. No adverse effects on heart rate or blood pressure were noted; however, fat oxidation did increase in certain individuals.

GREEN TEA

Green tea has achieved world-wide recognition for its numerous health benefits. It has been shown to lower cholesterol and blood pressure, protect against certain cancers, block bacteria and viruses, improve digestion and reduce the risk of ulcers and strokes. Green tea also helps to support weight loss. It provides a source of caffeine (approximately twenty to fifty milligrams per cup), a known thermogenic agent. Green tea is also rich in catechins, a type of antioxidant. In preliminary research, the combination of these ingredients has been found to help promote weight loss by burning more fat calories.

Research on Green Tea

There are a handful of studies that have evaluated the weight-loss potential of green tea. In 2002, researchers at the National Institute of Health and Medical Research in Marseille, France reported the results of a study of a green tea extract in seventy moderately obese adults (ninety percent women) ranging in age from twenty to sixty-nine years. The patients took a standardized green tea extract providing 375 milligrams of green tea catechins per day for three months. Waist circumference decreased by an average of 4.5 percent and body weight was reduced by an average of 4.6 percent.

Researchers at the University of Geneva studied the effects of green tea on energy expenditures (calorie burning) in a small group of ten healthy young men. For six weeks, the men took two capsules at each meal consisting of either green tea extract plus fifty milligrams of caffeine, only fifty milligrams of caffeine or a placebo. The participants followed a routine weight maintenance diet. Three times during the study, they spent twenty-four hours in a special room where their respiration and energy expenditures were measured. Energy expenditures were four percent higher for men taking green tea extract compared to those taking caffeine or placebo. They also found that men taking the green tea extract used more fat calories for energy than those taking placebo. There was no difference between the caffeine users and the placebo users in terms of either overall calorie burning or fat calorie burning. The researchers concluded that the benefits seen in the green tea group cannot be explained by caffeine intake alone. They suggested that the caffeine interacted with the flavonoids in green tea to alter the body's use of norepinephrine, a chemical transmitter in the nervous system, and to increase the rate of calorie burning. Green tea did not affect the heart rate in the study participants.

For those who are looking at the general health benefits of green tea, studies have found benefits with ranges between three and ten cups or more daily. Green tea can also be taken in capsule or tablet form. The usual recommended dosage is one tablet or capsule, three to four times daily, of a product that provides ninety milligrams of EGCG and fifty milligrams of caffeine per dosage. Although green tea is well tolerated, it should be used cautiously by those sensitive to caffeine, such as those with high blood pressure, kidney disease, insomnia or increased intraocular (eye) pressure.

Green tea may offer some additional benefits for weight management. Theanine, which is an amino acid present in green tea, has become a popular stress-reducing supplement. Studies conducted on Suntheanine® brand of theanine

WATCH THESE RISING STARS

Bitter melon (*Momordica charantia*) has been observed to have blood sugar lowering effects. This plant has been used for centuries in traditional Indian, Chinese and African pharmacopeia. Doctors in India are so confident of bitter melon's positive effect on diabetics, they dispense it in some of the most modern hospitals. People with Type 2 diabetes using bitter melon should be supervised by a qualified health care provider.

Chromium is an essential trace mineral found in a wide variety of foods. It is important in the burning of carbohydrates and fats in the body, and helps insulin do its work of making blood sugar (glucose, our basic fuel) available to cells. Chromium picolinate, a combination of the element chromium and picolinic acid, is a nutritional supplement that works to increase the efficiency of insulin to optimal levels. Combining chromium with picolinic acid simply aids in efficient chromium absorption.

Glucosol, extracted from banaba leaves (*Lagerstroemia speciosa*) contains corosolic acid. Also known as Crepe Myrtle, Queen's Flower or Pride of India, banaba has been one of the most effective plants used in Ayurvedic medicine for diabetes and weight control. It has been known to lower blood sugar levels in Type 2 diabetes.

Gymnema (*Gymnema sylvestre*) has been shown to lower fasting blood sugar levels and regenerate pancreatic cells that produce insulin (called islet cells. Gymnema enhances insulin's action, reduces fasting blood sugar levels (only in diabetics) and may stimulate islet cell regeneration.

Mulberry leaf extract (*Sucralite*™) has been shown in preliminary studies to help control blood sugar levels, decrease after-meal blood sugar levels in normal and diabetic people, and improve insulin secretion. This product works by inhibiting an enzyme called alpha-glucosidase, which is involved in sugar metabolism.

have found that it can promote calming and relaxation without causing sedation or memory loss, which can occur with prescription sedatives. Since stress raises cortisol, and elevated cortisol can lead to weight gain, this supplement may offer some benefits. Suntheanine may also be effective in curbing stress-related eating, such as cravings and binge eating, by modulating hormones. The recommended dosage is 50 to 200 milligrams twice or three times daily.

—⁓—

You should now have a greater understanding of the glycemic index, and the steps that need to be taken in order to achieve improved glycemic control and effective weight loss. I want to stress again that the glycemic index, while clinically proven to have merits for several health concerns, works best when combined with other lifestyle changes. Those changes include healthy food choices and portion sizes, regular exercise, a good night's rest, a stress management program and supplements. In Chapter 9 I outline my recommendations for taking everything you've learned and putting it into action.

9
CHAPTER

Putting It All Together

Give yourself a pat on the back. You now know more about why blood sugar management is important to overall health, and you understand the basic principles of eating low GI meals. Now, you are ready to put it all together in your day-to-day life. This won't be as hard as you may think. The most important thing is to hang in there during the transition from high GI foods to low GI foods.

STOCKING YOUR PANTRY

One of the biggest saboteurs of maintaining healthy eating habits is not having good food choices in the fridge when you're rushed, stressed and/or hungry. Instead of the traditional weekly bulk grocery shop, get into the habit of grocery shopping at least twice a week. Buy smaller amounts of foods, fresh fruits and vegetables and shop with certain meals in mind (this will help you steer clear of impulse purchases).

EVERYDAY BASICS

The following items are great for eating nutritiously every day:

- One percent dairy products or fortified soy beverages,
- Plain (unsweetened) yogurt,
- Eggs (organic, omega-3 are best)
- Whole-grain breads such as rye, sourdough, pita and flat bread, and
- Nuts and nut butters (almond and cashew).

FRUITS AND VEGETABLES

There are several strategies to increase your fresh produce consumption:

- Keep a ready supply of salad fixings: different lettuces, spinach, sprouts, tomatoes, carrots, celery, peppers, radishes, endive and cucumbers.
- Make sure you have at least three different vegetables in addition to what you might find in a salad (this includes asparagus, bok choy, kale or collard greens, green and yellow beans, snow peas or cauliflower). This way you can have a salad and a main vegetable as often as possible.

- Try yam, sweet potato or taro as a low GI substitute for potatoes.
- Select a variety of fruits, including berries, apples, oranges, pears, plums and grapefruit. Bananas, cherries, and melons have a higher GI value and should be eaten in smaller quantities.
- Try to squeeze in a lemon a day either as a flavor for meals or sliced in water.

FOR THE PANTRY

These staples are excellent to have on-hand:

- Whole-grain flour (whole wheat, rice bran and soy flour)
- Honey and pure maple syrup
- Whole-grain brown rice wild rice
- Whole wheat pasta
- Other grains such as quinoa, buckwheat and couscous
- Beans (try to pick up at least three or four different types with each grocery trip)
- Canned tomatoes, sugar-free tomato paste
- Canned salmon and tuna
- Low GI cereals (try different brands to see what you like; don't be afraid to combine low and moderate GI cereals)
- Low GI energy bars (for example Larabar®; eat only a couple each week)
- Slow-cooked oatmeal
- Extra virgin olive oil
- Dried spices
- Powdered cinnamon

IN THE FREEZER

Limit your intake of pre-packaged food, but stock frozen foods such as: berries, vegetables and lean meats such as chicken, turkey and fish.

SOMETHING SWEET, SOMETHING SALTY

There will always be times when you feel like something sweet or salty. You can enjoy a treat, just not everyday. Train yourself to reach for fresh or dried fruit to satisfy sweet cravings. For salt cravings, try a handful of nuts or seeds. When that just doesn't do the trick, consider a small portion of dark chocolate with vanilla frozen yogurt or baked apples with cinnamon sprinkled on top, or blue corn chips with hummus or feta dip. If you'd really like to have the double-fudge, chocolate piece-of-heaven cake, take a small portion and enjoy. You can also experiment with different recipes to find a low GI variation to your favourite dessert. You may find as your body becomes accustomed to low GI meals, that high GI foods just don't make you feel well. As a result, your desire for indulgence foods decrease with time.

Seven-day GI Meal Suggestions

Use the chart on the following page as an example of a 7-day low GI meal plan. Create meals that combine a low GI carb with protein and healthy fats, and vegetables or fruit. Drink up to eight glasses of pure water each day and remember to include herbal or green tea.

Holiday and Restaurant Survival Strategies

Following the glycemic index does not mean you've had your last meal at a restaurant or holiday feast. It's quite the opposite. Many diets are restrictive, which often results in binge eating. With the GI, you can continue to enjoy a variety of foods at home or in restaurant but don't forget to make good low GI choices and create balanced meals.

Here are some points to consider regarding restaurants and holidays:

1. Have a light, low GI snack before you head out to a dinner party or restaurant so that you aren't tempted by high GI appetizers.
2. Choose restaurants that you know offer a variety of freshly prepared foods. Avoid fast food.
3. Consider trying new foods. Many foods from Indian, Thai, Greek and Japanese restaurants are naturally lower GI.
4. Don't be shy to ask questions. If you feel embarrassed, tell the waiter you are diabetic to ease the tension.
5. If you can't find a low GI meal to your liking, order a half-portion of the meal you would like, or see if the chef will make you a special dish.
6. Avoid ordering an appetizer, unless it's a green salad with a low GI dressing, grilled vegetables or broiled scallops or shrimps.
7. Limit alcohol consumption to no more than two glasses and drink plenty of water with lemon.
8. Choose to have either a glass of wine, whole wheat bread or dessert but not all three. If you choose to have bread, make sure your main meal is primarily protein and vegetables. If you choose to have dessert, ask the chef which dessert is most appropriate for a low GI diet.
9. If you are at a restaurant that serves large portions, ask for a take-out container when you order so that you don't overeat.
10. To lower the GI of foods such as pasta, baked potatoes or rice, you can open a capsule of Phase 2 and sprinkle it on the food before you eat.

When planning holiday meals don't be a slave to tradition, especially if traditional foods make you feel unwell. While there might be some temporary taste bud satisfaction, what counts is how you feel afterward. If what you eat haunts you afterward, either through indigestion or guilt, you should not be eating those foods. Instead, have fun creating your own holiday menu that includes fresh

	Sunday	Monday	Tuesday	Wednesday	Thursday	Friday	Saturday
Breakfast	two poached or scrambled eggs, turkey bacon, and one slice of pumpernickel or rye toast	low GI cereal such as oatmeal or All-Bran, skim or soy milk, and half a banana	½ cantaloupe, with sliced pears and plums, one low GI energy bar (Larabar)	whole-grain toast with mustard, one slice of one percent cheese, sautéed mushrooms and tomato	power shake: blend one scoop of protein powder, with water, milk or soy milk, ice cubes and berries	one cup of plain yogurt with strawberries, two tablespoons ground flax or hemp and s prinkled with cinnamon	two whole wheat pancakes with a teaspoon of real maple syrup, and ½ cup of raspberries
Snack	a cup of plain yogurt with blueberries	one stalk of celery with one boiled egg (chopped)	½ cup of chick peas with orange and red pepper slices	¼ cup of almonds and an apple	a low GI energy bar	an orange or ½ cup of cherries	one percent cottage cheese with cucumber slices
Lunch	one slice of pizza made with whole wheat crust, one percent cheese and chicken	crustless quiche made with whole grain flour, turkey and broccoli	lentil soup with corn tortilla and mixed greens	salmon sandwich on whole wheat pita bread with lettuce and tomatoes	egg salad in lettuce wrap with tomato and cucumber salad	hummus with flat bread, alfalfa sprouts	whole wheat pasta with beans and eggplant
Snack	carrot and celery sticks with yogurt dip	an apple with its skin	¼ cup of almonds	red grapes	dried apricots	½ cup trail mix	an apple with slice of one percent cheese
Dinner	green salad, long-grain brown and wild rice with zucchini, onion and grilled salmon, bok choy or swiss chard	green salad, sweet potato, with turkey breast and green and yellow beans	green salad, shrimp and scallops with whole-grain pasta (cooked al dente) and asparagus	green salad, vegetarian chili served on cauliflower mash with snow peas	green salad, grilled salmon with lemon, yellow squash and one small whole grain bun	green salad, chicken with turkey bacon and avocado, on a bed of cooked spinach	green salad, small steak, ½ cup canned beets and flat bread

takes on classic dishes. For example, substitute cauliflower or sweet potato mash instead of mashed potato, and instead of gravy thickened with corn starch, reach for different flavours of mustard and fresh or dried herbs. If you are dining at a friend's house and are concerned there won't be food choices for you, simply bring what you need.

Another concern with restaurant and holiday meals is that they often break the cycle of healthy eating habits. For people who struggle to establish consistent healthy eating habits, a break in the routine can be damaging on a larger scale, making it harder to get back on-track. If you know this to be true about yourself, work hard to incorporate healthy GI choices at every meal. You will feel so proud of yourself and it will make it that much easier to continue on your path to success.

Brace for Impact

Be prepared for some rocky roads during the transition to low GI foods. While in only a short period of time you should start feel better, most notably with more balanced mood, increased energy and better digestion, you could also have some temporary side effects from the change of diet. These side effects might include headaches, fatigue, irritability and cravings. This is your body telling you that it wants a blood sugar boost NOW. If you are going to overcome food cravings and take control of your blood sugar, you are going to have to suffer through these difficult times. (However, please consult your physician if these side effects last longer than a week.) If you can make it through the transition period and get your diet on the right track, with balanced blood sugar instead of blood sugar highs and lows, you will begin to feel well, energized and more in control of what you eat. In the meantime, reach for an apple, an orange pepper, a small amount of dried fruit and nuts, or yogurt and berries.

You may also feel self-conscious about being a "high-maintenance" or "fussy eater." In some cases, co-workers, friends or family may make unkind comments about your new habits. You may experience some peer pressure to not "rock the boat" and to eat what everyone else is eating. Take heart. This just comes with the territory of eating outside the traditional diet, so you better learn to ignore it. What you need to remember is that nobody else is living your life. You have only one chance and you need to make the most of it, and that includes feeling your best everyday. Obesity and diabetes can make you feel lousy and take years off your life. Remind yourself of the end goal when you're faced with insensitive comments—just smile to yourself and shrug them off, knowing you are doing what's best for your health.

Making it Stick

To make this whole process worthwhile, you're going to want to see results. Long-term results take work but they will come with five rules of thumb:

1. Eat a balanced diet with a variety of foods everyday. Food is not the enemy so experiment and have fun creating a new menu of low GI, balanced meals. Take cooking classes and learn to love food again, without the guilt.

2. Watch your portion sizes and don't overdo it at any given meal. Since you will never again need to be restrictive, you know that there will be many satisfying meals each day of your future. If you do indulge in high GI foods once in a while, eat small amounts and don't punish yourself afterward.

3. Be physically active at least five days a week, every week. Don't make excuses not to exercise, instead tell yourself reasons why you like to exercise—more energy, better sleep, and a better mood. If weather conditions are keeping you indoors, turn on the radio or put in a CD and dance or skip.

4. Be smart about your supplements. Choose clinically-tested supplements to support your blood sugar management and weight-loss efforts, such as fiber, Phase 2 and CLA.

5. Make an effort to have a positive attitude and to be kind to yourself. This is the hardest of all because typically people with weight or health problems feel like the deck is stacked against them. They can feel overwhelmed by negative thoughts. Work hard to overcome negative thinking and celebrate every success, especially during the transition. You might create a weekly reward system for yourself (not with food). Each week you maintain your diet and exercise routine, treat yourself to something very special. You will have earned it.

—〰—

An English proverb says, "Don't dig your own grave with a knife and fork." I believe that now is the time to make the change to a low GI diet. The glycemic index offers us a greater understanding of the role of carbohydrates and how to make better choices in our daily eating habits. Improving our eating habits is the long-term answer to many health concerns we face as a result of our diet, especially obesity and diabetes. This health-conscious eating style has proven benefits for weight loss, appetite control and blood sugar management. Furthermore, the secondary result from this sensible plan, which includes an emphasis on eating whole-grains, legumes, nuts and assorted vegetables and fruits, is the reduced risk of chronic disease such as cardiovascular disease.

A low GI diet can be easily implemented into your home without having to cook separate meals for different family members. It poses no health risks, making it a safe choice for children, teenagers, pregnant women and nursing moms, seniors and those with existing health concerns (food allergies aside). It is my sincere hope that you are able to take what you've learned from this book and put it into action in your life. I am confident that if you put the time and effort into following a low GI diet, combined with regular exercise and proper sleep and stress management strategies, you are sure to see tremendous results for your overall health. I wish you the best of luck as you set forth on your path to weight loss success.

Resources and References

RECOMMENDED READING

The Natural Fat-Loss Pharmacy by Harry Preuss. Broadway, 2007.

Beyond the Basics from the Canadian Diabetes Association, 2006.

The Path to Phenomenal Health by Sam Graci. Wiley, 2005.

The Low GI Diet Revolution by Dr. Jennie Brand-Miller and Kaye Foster-Powell with Joanna McMillan-Price. Marlowe and Company, 2005.

Cracking the Metabolic Code by Dr. James B. LaValle. Basic Health Publications, 2004.

How to Prevent and Treat Diabetes with Natural Medicine by Michael Murray ND. Riverhead Books, 2004.

The Body Sense Natural Diet by Lorna Vanderhaeghe, John Wiley & Sons, 2004

Leslie Beck's 10 Steps to Healthy Eating by Leslie Beck, RN. Viking Canada, 2002.

Fat Wars by Brad King, John Wiley & Sons Canada, 2000.

HELPFUL RESOURCES

For information on the glycemic index and healthy eating:
University of Sydney, official site of the Glycemic Index:
www.glycemicindex.com

Glycemic Research Institute: www.glycemic.com
Harvard School of Public Health, The Nutrition Source: www.hsph.harvard.edu/nutritionsource

For information on diabetes:
Canadian Diabetes Association: www.diabetes.ca
American Diabetes Association: www.diabetes.org
Diabetes UK: www.diabetes.org/uk
International Diabetes Institute (Australia): www.diabetes.com.au

For general information on herbs, vitamins and nutritional supplements:
www.healthwell.com
www.pdrhealth.com
www.wholehealthmd.com
www.iherb.com
Linus Pauling Institute: lpi.oregonstate.edu

For eating disorders information:
National Eating Disorder Information Centre: www.nedic.ca
The Renfrew Center Foundation: www.renfrew.org
The Cedric Centre for Wellness: www.compulsiveeating.com

For information on the products discussed in this book:
Phase 2 Starch Neutralizer: www.phase2info.com
PGX: www.slimstyles.com
Tonalin CLA: www.tonalin.com
Advantra Z: www.nutratechinc.com

Other Health Links:
Author's website: www.sherrytorkos.com
American College of Sports Medicine: http://acsm.org/index.asp
American Heart Association Fitness Resource: www.justmove.org
Centers for Disease Control and Prevention: www.cdc.gov
The Mayo Clinic: www.mayoclinic.com
The Institute of Medicine: www.iom.edu
National Institutes of Health: www.nih.gov
National Institutes of Health, Calculate your BMI; www.nhlbisupport.com/bmi/
Reuters Health (for the latest medical and healthcare news): www.reutershealth.com
Web MD: www.webmd.com

PRODUCT DIRECTORY:

The supplements for weight loss and blood sugar control listed in this book are available under the following brands:

PHASE 2®

BodySense® Natural Diet Program by Preferred Nutrition
CARB CUTTER® Phase 2™ by Health & Nutrition Systems International, Inc.
METASlim Carb Neutralizer & Fat Blocker, METASlim Phase 2®, and METASlim
   Kit by WN Pharmaceuticals® Ltd.
Phase 2® by Nature's Harmony®, NOW® Foods, and Vivitas™
Slenderite™ and Carb Intercept® by Natrol®
Total Lean Advance™ by General Nutrition Centers Inc.
TRIMSPA® CarbSpa by Nutramerica Corporation

TONALIN® CLA

Tonalin® CLA is available by Country Life®, General Nutrition Centers Inc., Jarrow
Formulas®, Natrol®, Natural Factors®, Nature's Bounty®, Nature's Way®, Preferred
   Nutrition®, and WN Pharmaceuticals® Ltd.

ADVANTRA Z®

Green Tea Fat Burner® by Applied Nutrition®
Bitter Orange by Nature's Way®
Cortislim® Original™ and Cortislim® Burn™ by Window Rock Enterprises, Inc.
Diet Fuel® and Ripped Fuel® by Twin Lab®
Lean System 7® by iSotori
Look Slim by Prolab®

PGX™

Slim styles™ by Natural Factors®
METAslim No Nonsense Diet™ by WN Pharmaceuticals® Ltd.
BodySense® Meal Replacement with PGX® by Preferred Nutrition

REFERENCES:

Augustin LS, Galeone C, Dal Maso L, et al. Glycemic index, glycemic load and risk of prostate cancer. *Int J Cancer* 2004;112:446.

Ballerini, R. Evaluation of efficacy and safety of a food supplement for weight control through the reduced calories-intake from carbohydrates vs. placebo. Data on file. Pharmachem Laboratories, Kearny, New Jersey, 2002.

Bell SJ, Sears B. Low-glycemic-load diets: impact on obesity and chronic diseases. *Crit Rev Food Sci Nutr*. 2003;43(4):357-77.

Birmingham CL, Muller JL, Palepn A, Spinelli JJ, Anise AH: Cost of obesity in Canada. *CMAJ* 1999;160: 483-488.

Blankson H, Stakkestad JA, Fagertun H, et al. Conjugated linoleic acid reduces body fat mass in overweight and obese humans. *J Nutr* 2000;130(12):2943-8.

Boule NG, Haddad E, Kenny GP, Wells GA, Sigal RJ. Effects of exercise on glycemic control and body mass in type 2 diabetes mellitus: a meta-analysis of controlled clinical trials. *JAMA* 2001;286(10):1218-27.

Brehm BJ, Seeley RJ, Daniels SR, et al. A Randomized Trial Comparing a Very Low Carbohydrate Diet and a Calorie-Restricted Low Fat Diet on Body Weight and Cardiovascular Risk Factors in Healthy Women. *J Clin Endocrinol Metab* 2003 Apr;88(4):1617-23.

Carmona, Richard H. M.D., M.P.H., F.A.C.S., Surgeon General, U.S. Public Health Service, U.S. Department of Health and Human Services. Statements made before the Subcommittee on Competition, Infrastructure, and Foreign Commerce Committee on Commerce, Science, and Transportation United States Senate, released March 2, 2004.

Chantre P and Lairon D. Recent findings of green tea extract AR25 (Exolise) and its activity for the treatment of obesity. *Phytomedicine* 2002; 9:3-8.

Chaoyang L, Ford ES, Mokdad AH, et al. Recent Trends in Waist Circumference and Waist-Height Ratio Among US Children and Adolescents. *Pediatrics* 2006;118: e1391-e1398.

Colker CM, et al. Effects of Citrus aurantium extract, caffeine, and St. John's wort on body fat loss, lipid levels, and mood states in overweight healthy adults. *Curr Ther Res* 1999;60:145-153.

Cunningham Dr. Sam, et al. "Managing Glycemic Response" *Nutraceuticals World*. 20/09/2006.

Dansinger ML, Gleason JL, Griffith JL, et al. One Year Effectiveness of the Atkins, Ornish, Weight Watchers, and Zone Diets in Decreasing Body Weight and Heart Disease Risk. Presented at the American Heart Association Scientific Sessions November 12, 2003 in Orlando, Florida.

DeLany JP, Blohm E, Truett AA, et al. Conjugated linoleic acid rapidly reduces body fat content in mice without affecting energy intake. *Am J Physiol* 1999; 276: 1172-1179.

Dulloo AG, et al. The thermogenic properties of ephedrine/methylxantine mixtures 11: human studies. *Int J Obes* 1986; 10:467-481.

Dulloo AG, Duret C, Rohrer D, et al. Efficacy of a green tea extract rich in catechin polyphenols and caffeine in increasing 24-h energy expenditure and fat oxidation in humans. *Am J Clin Nutr* 1999;70:1040-5.

Flier JS. "Obesity". In Joslin's Diabetes Mellitus, edited by R. C Kahn and G. C. Weir. 13th ed. Philadelphia: Lea & Febiger. 1994. 351-61.

Foster GD, Wyatt HR, Hill JO, et al. A Randomized Trial of a Low-Carbohydrate Diet for Obesity. *N Engl J Med* 2003;348(21)2082-2090.

Foster-Powell K, Holt SH, Brand-Miller JC. International table of glycemic index and glycemic load values: 2002. *Am J Clin Nut*. 2002;76:5-56.

Franz MJ, Bantle JP, Beebe CA, Evidence-based nutrition principles and recommendations for the treatment and prevention of diabetes and related complications. *Diabetes Care* 2002;148-98 .

Gaullier JM, Halse J, Hoye K, et al. Conjugated linoleic acid supplementation for 1 y reduces body fat mass in healthy overweight humans. *Am J Clin Nutr* 2004;79:1118-25.

Haffner SM. Epidemiological studies on the effects of hyperglycemia and improvement of glycemic control on macrovascular events in type 2 diabetes. *Diabetes Care* 1999; 22 Suppl 3:54-56.

Health Canada. Canadian Community Health Survey, 2004. Accessed November 23, 2006. Available online at http://www.hc-sc.gc.ca/fn-an/surveill/nutrition/commun/index_e.html

Higginbotham S, Zhang ZF, Lee IM, Cook NR, Buring JE, Liu S. Dietary glycemic load and breast cancer risk in the Women's Health Study. *Cancer Epidemiol Biomarkers Prev* 2004;13(1):65-70.

Higginbotham S, Zhang ZF, Lee IM, et al. Dietary glycemic load and risk of colorectal cancer in the Women's Health Study. *J Natl Cancer Inst* 2004;96(3):229-233.

Institute of Medicine of the National Academies. Dietary Reference Intakes for Energy, Carbohydrate, Fiber, Fat, Fatty Acids, Cholesterol, Protein, and Amino Acids. Accessed October 24, 2006. Available online at: www.iom.edu

Jenkins DJ, Kendall CW, Augustin LS, et al. Glycemic index: overview of implications in health and disease. *Am J Clin Nutr* 2002;76:266S-73S.

King AC, et al. Moderate-intensity exercise and self-rated quality of sleep in older adults: a randomized controlled trial. *JAMA* 1997;277:32-37.

Kings Fund Policy Institute. Counting the Cost: The Real Impact of Non-Insulin Dependent Diabetes. A Kings Fund Report Commissioned by The British Diabetic Association, London, 1996.

Kramer F.M., et al. Long-term follow-up of behavioural treatment of obesity: Patterns of regain among men and women. *Intl J Obesity* 1989;13:123-126.

Kushi LH, Fee RM, Folsom AR, et al. Physical activity and mortality in postmenopausal women. *JAMA* 1997;277(16):1287-92.

Lean ME, et al. Waist Circumference as a measure for indicating need for weight management. *BMJ* 1995; 311:158-161.

Lehrer S, Diamond EJ, Stagger S, et al. Serum insulin level, disease stage, prostate specific antigen (PSA) and Gleason score in prostate cancer. *Br J Cancer* 2002;87(7):726-8.

Liese AD, Roach AK, Sparks KC, et al. Whole-grain intake and insulin sensitivity: the Insulin Resistance Atherosclerosis Study. *Am J Clin Nutr* 2003; 78:965-71.

Ludwig DS. Dietary glycemic index and obesity. *J Nutr* 2000:130:280S-283S.

Ludwig DS, Majzoub Joseph A, Al-Zahrani Ahmed et al. High glycemic index foods, overeating and obesity. *Pediatrics* 1999;103(3):e26.

Lynch J, et al. Moderately intense physical activities and high levels of cardio-respiratory fitness reduce the risk of non-insulin-dependent diabetes mellitus in middle-aged men. *Arch Intern Med* 1996;156:1307-1314.

MacDonald HB. Conjugated linoleic acid and disease prevention: a review of current knowledge. *J Am Coll Nutr* 2000;19(2):11S-118S.

Madrick B. Canadian Diabetes Association. "Carbohydrate Counting." Canadian Diabetes Association. 16 June 2002.

Manson JE, et al. Body Weight and Mortality. *N Engl J Med* 1995;333:677-85.

McMillan-Price J, Petocz P, Atkinson F, et al. Comparison of 4 diets of varying glycemic load on weight loss and cardiovascular risk reduction in overweight and obese young adults: a randomised controlled trial. *Arch Intern Med.* 2006;166:1466-1475.

Mendis Shanthi et al. "Integrated Management of Cardiovascular Risk" Report of a WHO (World Health Organization) meeting, Geneva July 2002.

Michaud DS, Liu S, Giovannucci E, Willett WC, Colditz GA, Fuchs CS. Dietary sugar, glycemic load, and pancreatic cancer risk in a prospective study. *J Natl Cancer Inst* 2002;94(17):1293-1300.

Mokdad AH, Bowman BA, Ford ES, Vinicor F, Marks JS, Koplan JP. The continuing epidemics of obesity and diabetes in the United States. *JAMA* 2001;286(10):1195-2000.

National Institute of Diabetes and Digestive and Kidney Diseases. Understanding Adult Obesity. NIH Publ. No. 94-3680. Rockville, MD: National Institutes of Health, 1993.

National Institutes of Health. Consensus conference on methods for voluntary weight loss and control. *Ann Int Med* 1992;116:942-49.

North American Society for the Study of Obesity's Annual Scientific Meeting, Las Vegas, Nov. 14-18, 2004. WebMD Medical News: "Sleep More and You May Control Eating More." WebMD Medical News: "Why Dieting Makes You Hungrier." News release, North American Society for the Study of Obesity.

Organization for Economic Co-Operation and Development (OECD) Health Data 2006: a comparative analysis of 30 countries. Accessed November 23, 2006. Available online http://www.oecd.org/health/healthdata/

Organization for Economic Co-Operation and Development (OECD). "Obesity and Health Forum 2004" Presented by John P. Martin May 12, 2004.

Office of the Surgeon General, "Overweight and Obesity: The Surgeon General's Call To Action To Prevent and Decrease Overweight and Obesity", December, 2001. Accessed November 23, 2006. Available online at: http://www.surgeongeneral.gov/topics/obesity

Park Y, Albright KJ, Storkson JM, et al. Changes in body composition in mice during feeding and withdrawal of conjugated linoleic acid. *Lipids* 1998;34(3):243-248.

Park Y, Albright KJ, Liu W, et al. Effect of conjugated linoleic acid on body composition in mice. *Lipids* 1997;32(8):853-858.

Pelkman CL. Effects of the glycemic index of foods on serum concentrations of high-density lipoprotein cholesterol and triglycerides. *Curr Atherscler Rep* 2001;3(6):456-61.

Pereira MA, Liu S. Types of carbohydrates and risk of cardiovascular disease. *J Womens Health* 2003;12:115-22.

Pi-Sunyer FX, et al: Medical hazards of obesity. *Ann Intern Med* 1993;119:655-660.

Reaven G. The insulin resistance syndrome: past, present, and future. Presented at The First Annual World Congress on the Insulin Resistance Syndrome; November 20-22, 2003; Los Angeles, California.

Riserus, U, Berglund L, Vessby B. Conjugated linoleic acid (CLA) reduced abdominal adipose tissue in obese middle-aged men with signs of the metabolic syndrome: a randomised controlled trial. *Int J Obes Relat Metab Disord* 2001 Aug;25(8):1129-35.

Shrier I. Stretching before exercise: an evidence based approach. *Br J Sports Med* 2000;34(5):324-5.

Schulze MB, Liu S, Rimm EB, et al. Glycemic index, glycemic load, and dietary fiber intake and incidence of type 2 diabetes in younger and middle-aged women. *Am J Clin Nutr* 2004;80:348-56.

Silvera SA, Jain M, Howe GR, Miller AB, Rohan TE. Dietary carbohydrates and breast cancer risk: a prospective study of the roles of overall glycemic index and glycemic load. *Int J Cancer* 2005;114(4):653-658.

Smedman A, Vessby B. Conjugated linoleic acid supplementation in humans—metabolic effects. *Lipids* 2001;36(8):773-81.

Steinberger J, Daniels SR. Obesity, Insulin Resistance, Diabetes, and Cardiovascular Risk in Children. *Circulation* 2003;107:1448.

Thom E: A pilot study with the aim of studying the efficacy and tolerability of Tonalin CLA on the body composition in humans. Medstat Research, Ltd., of Lillestrom, Norway, 1997.

Van Gaal LF, Mertens IL, Ballaux D. What is the relationship between risk factor reduction and degree of weight loss? *Eur Heart J Suppl* 2005;7(50):L21-L26.

Wolever TM, Yang M, Zeng XY, et al. Food glycemic index, as given in glycemic index tables, a significant determinant of glycemic responses ellicited by composit breakfast meals. *Am J Clin Nutr* 2006;83:1306-1312.